CW01497169

# LIVE TO EAT

## EMILY ENGLISH

Also by Emily English

**SO GOOD**

# LIVE TO EAT

## EMILY ENGLISH

**The food you crave, the nutrition you need**

SEVEN DIALS

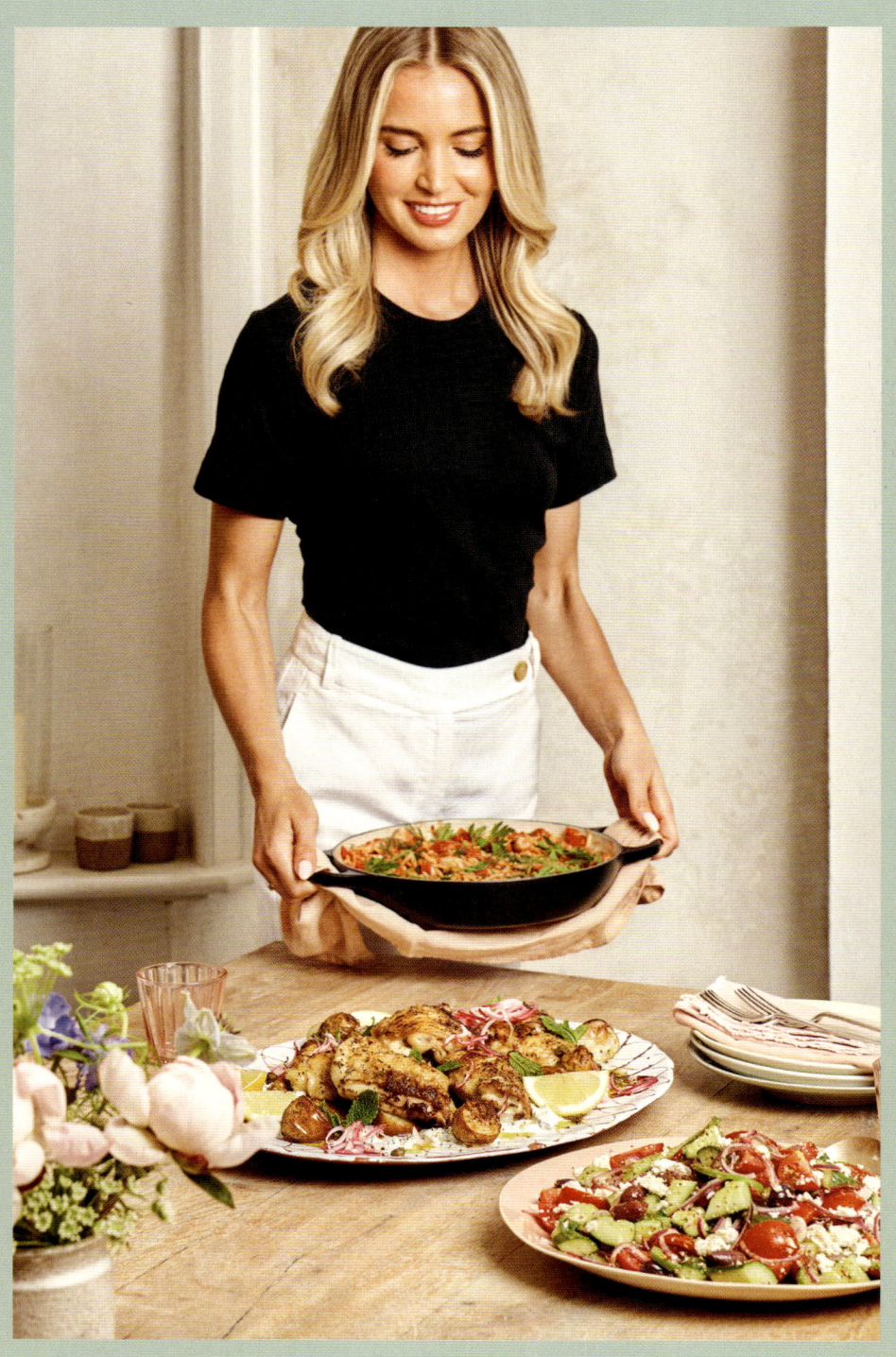

# CONTENTS

# Introduction

# Live to Eat: What It Means to Me

When I think of the title of this book, *Live to Eat*, it's more than just a phrase to me – it's an ethos, a way of life and an overarching philosophy that has shaped everything I do both in and out of the kitchen. It's about celebrating food, loving every bite and understanding that healthy eating doesn't have to mean sacrificing incredible flavours or joyful dishes. Eating well should be something we can look forward to, not a monotonous chore we dread. I truly believe that good nutrition and delicious food can and *should* go hand in hand.

Growing up, food in my family was never something to be feared or restricted. My first job as a child was in my granny's restaurant kitchen, observing the magic of cooking and learning about ingredients and combinations to create dishes that brought smiles to people's faces. Food was her way of life, her language of love, and I still take so much inspiration from her in what I do today. Having a heavy interest in science, I was also fascinated by the inner workings of the body and how what we eat can affect everything from our energy levels to our gut health and our overall well-being. That combination of curiosity for what was on my plate and what was happening inside me was the start of my journey.

But there was a time when my relationship with food became complicated. After a period in the modelling industry, food started to feel like the enemy – something I had to control rather than enjoy. It was during this time that I realised how much misinformation was out there about nutrition, and how damaging a negative relationship with food could be. That's what pushed me to leave the modelling behind and pursue something that I truly loved and had a passion for. So I studied

# 'I want you to feel inspired, not restricted, when you think about food'

nutrition at university, to dive deeper into the science of food, and to learn how to nourish the body properly *without* losing the sense of joy that food should rightfully bring.

So when I say *Live to Eat,* I mean embracing food as a source of pleasure, with its ability to fuel and nourish all at once. I want to help people understand that food isn't just about calories, nutrients or 'good' versus 'bad'. It's about balance, enjoyment and creating a sustainable, healthy relationship with what's on your plate. I absolutely love food, and I don't believe that good nutrition should ever come at the cost of flavour.

My mission with this book – and with everything I do, really – is to show that healthy eating doesn't have to feel like deprivation. You don't have to give up your favourite meals or settle for bland, dull 'health food'. With the right approach, eating well can be the most satisfying part of your day. I want you to feel inspired, not restricted, when you think about food. I want you to look forward to every meal, knowing that what you're eating is good for your body *and* for your soul.

Because, at the end of the day, we all deserve to enjoy our food. After all, we don't just eat to live – we live to eat.

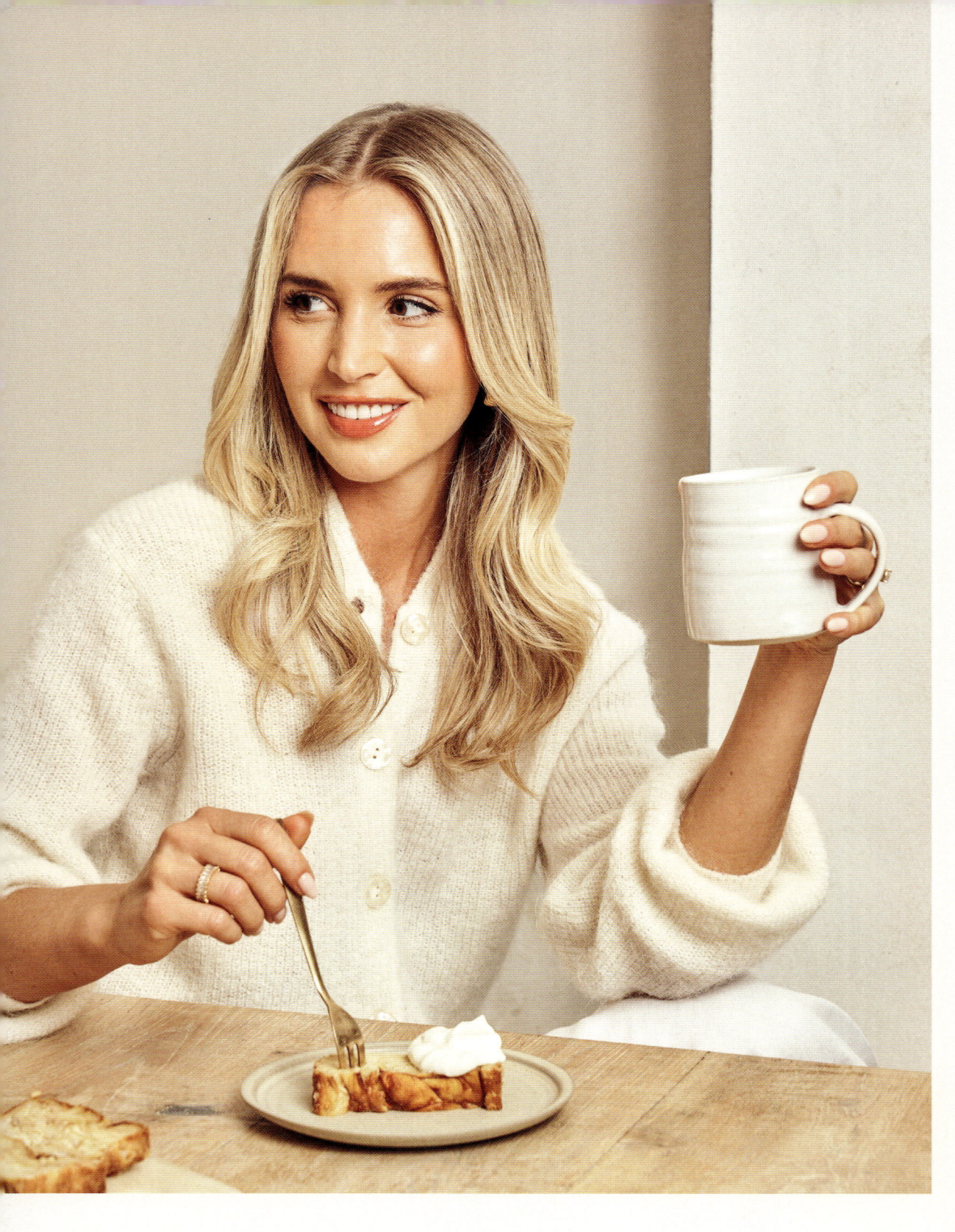

# Nutritional Information: What's Important and What's Not?

When it comes to making sense of nutritional information, it can be easy to feel lost in a sea of confusing numbers and terms – calories, protein, carbohydrates, sugar, fat, saturated fat, fibre, salt... But don't worry, you don't need a degree in nutritional science to understand the basics. Let's break it down simply and sensibly, so you know what really matters when you're looking at food labels.

## CALORIES: ENERGY IN, ENERGY OUT

Calories are a measure of energy, and your body needs energy to function; from walking and thinking to digesting and repairing, everything you do uses energy. However, while calories tell you how much energy is in your food, they don't tell you how balanced or nutritious that food is for you.

What's more important is where these calories come from. For example, 400 calories from a homemade meal with protein, vegetables and whole grains will be digested differently and benefit your body a lot more than 400 calories from a processed snack full of sugar and refined carbs. So yes, calories matter – but they're just part of the picture. Try not to be over-fixated with them; your body isn't a straight-up maths equation.

## PROTEIN: THE SECRET TO FEELING FULLER FOR LONGER

Protein is one of my favourite macronutrients. It's responsible for building and repairing tissues in your body, from muscles to skin, and even your hair and nails. But it's not just about maintenance – protein also plays a big role in how you feel after eating a meal. It's one of the most *satiating* nutrients, meaning it helps you feel fuller for longer, which can prevent cravings and manage hunger.

The reason protein helps you feel fuller for longer comes down to a few key factors: it has the ability to increase satiety hormones, slow down digestion and stabilise blood sugar levels, because it requires more energy for digestion. Together, these effects help prolong the feeling of fullness and provide a steady source of energy, making protein one of the most important nutrients to include in a balanced, satisfying diet.

Whether you get your protein from lean meats, fish, eggs, dairy or plant-based sources like beans and lentils, aim to include some with every meal.

## CARBOHYDRATES: ENERGY FOR LIFE BUT BALANCE IS KEY

Carbs have developed a bit of a bad reputation, but they're actually your body's main source of energy (your brain loves them!). The key is choosing the *right* types of carbohydrates – prioritising those from whole grains, vegetables, fruits and pulses, rather than the refined carbs in white bread, pastries and sugary snacks.

There are two types of carbohydrates: simple and complex. Simple carbs (like sugar) are digested quickly and can cause spikes in blood sugar, while complex carbs (like oats, wholegrain rice and sweet potatoes) are broken down more slowly, providing you with steady energy throughout the day.

## SUGAR: BALANCE, NOT ELIMINATION

Sugar has been heavily demonised in recent years, but in the context of a balanced diet, moderate amounts are not going to harm your health. While excessive sugar intake – particularly from highly processed foods

# 'It's not about demonising single ingredients, but about looking at the bigger picture'

and sugary drinks – can lead to health issues, it's important to remember that diet context is everything. Occasional sugar as part of a diet rich in wholefoods, fibre, protein and healthy fats isn't damaging.

It's not about demonising single ingredients, but about looking at the bigger picture of your overall diet. The key is balance, not elimination, and making mindful choices that fit into a sustainable, healthy lifestyle.

## FAT: THE GOOD, THE BAD AND WHY IT MATTERS

Fat is so often misunderstood. Despite what fad-diet culture may tell you, fat is not your enemy. In fact, healthy fats (like the unsaturated fats found in olive oil, avocados, nuts and seeds) are important for your body to function properly; they help absorb essential vitamins like A, D, E and K, and support brain and heart health.

I like to focus primarily on unsaturated fats and reduce my intake of saturated fats, which are often found in ultra-processed foods. Excessive consumption of saturated fats can raise cholesterol levels and increase the risk of heart disease, so moderation is key here.

## FIBRE: THE UNSUNG HERO

Fibre is one of the most important (yet often overlooked) nutrients. It helps support your gut microbiome, improves digestion, keeps you feeling fuller for longer and can even lower cholesterol levels. There are two kinds of fibre to be aware of: soluble and insoluble. Soluble fibre (found in oats, beans and apples) helps regulate blood sugar and reduce cholesterol, while insoluble fibre (found in whole grains and vegetables) helps to keep everything moving smoothly through your digestive system.

Most of us could do with eating more fibre – we should be aiming for around 30 grams of fibre per day, but many people don't get there. Aim to include a variety of fibre-rich foods like vegetables, fruits, whole grains and pulses in your diet. Not only will this help with digestion, but it's great for long-term heart and gut health.

## TO SUMMARISE . . .

When it comes to nutrition, we often get too fixated on individual nutrients like calories, carbs or fat, but good health is about more than just numbers. It's the *combination* of nutrients, the *consistency* of your eating habits and your overall *diet* patterns that really matter. It's about focusing on whole, minimally processed foods and aiming for balance. Instead of obsessing over single nutrients, pay attention to the bigger picture: eating a variety of nutrient-rich foods regularly for long-term health and well-being.

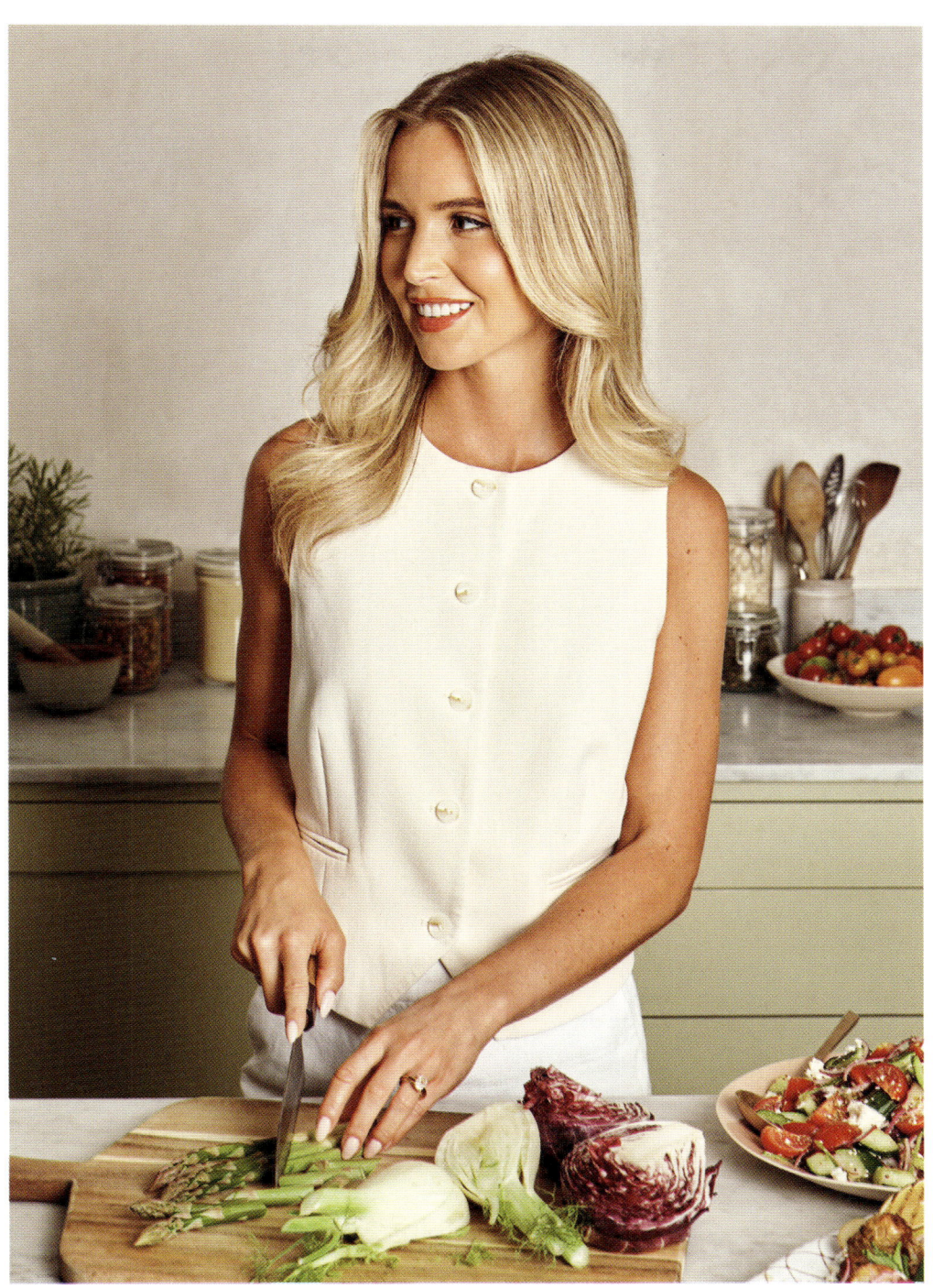

# Tips Beyond Food

When we talk about health and nutrition, it's easy to focus solely on what's on our plates, but true well-being goes far beyond food. Factors like sleep, stress, and even the language we use around food and ourselves all play a huge role in shaping our health and mindset. Here are some key non-food-related tips to help you achieve balance in your life:

## 1. PRIORITISE SLEEP

Good nutrition means little if you're running on empty. Sleep is when your body repairs and regenerates, and it's essential for everything from maintaining a healthy weight to managing stress and supporting cognitive functions.

Sleep is critical – not just for rest and recovery but for how your body regulates hunger and hormones. A lack of sleep can disrupt hormones like ghrelin and leptin, which control hunger and fullness. When you're sleep-deprived, ghrelin (the hunger hormone) increases, while leptin (the hormone that signals you're full) decreases, making you feel hungrier and more likely to crave sugary foods the next day.

Aim for seven to nine hours of quality sleep each night. Establishing a good bedtime routine – like reducing screen time before bed, keeping your room cool and dark, and sticking to a regular sleep schedule – can greatly improve your rest and recovery.

## 2. MANAGE STRESS

Stress has a direct impact on your overall health and eating habits. When you're stressed your body releases cortisol, a hormone that in short bursts helps you respond to immediate challenges. However, chronic stress keeps cortisol levels elevated, which can lead to increased appetite – especially for high-sugar, high-fat foods – as your body seeks quick energy sources to cope with the perceived threat.

Managing stress is crucial for maintaining balance in your diet and overall health. Stress-reducing activities like meditation, mindfulness, yoga or even just regular movement can help lower cortisol levels. Studies have also shown that practising mindfulness can reduce emotional eating and improve your relationship with food. Making time for self-care, hobbies and relaxation is just as important as making healthy food choices. Reducing stress not only benefits your mental health but can also prevent the hormonal triggers that lead to your food choices.

## 3. CHANGE THE LANGUAGE YOU USE AROUND FOOD AND YOUR BODY

How we talk about food and our bodies can significantly affect our relationship with them. Instead of labelling foods as 'good' or 'bad', think about food as our life source – something that nourishes, energises and supports us. Likewise, try to avoid using negative self-talk like 'I was bad today' or 'I deserve a treat'. These phrases can reinforce guilt or an all-or-nothing mindset around eating. Start speaking to yourself with kindness and balance – treat food and your body with respect and appreciate the role they play in your overall well-being.

Be kind to yourself. Health is a journey, not a destination. There will be ups and downs, and that's completely normal. Practising gratitude for what your body can do, rather than focusing on perceived flaws, can help shift your mindset. Likewise, give yourself grace when things don't go perfectly – whether that's an indulgent meal, a missed workout or a stressful day. Balance is about flexibility, not perfection.

## 4. MOVEMENT BEYOND THE GYM

Movement is unique to each of us, and it's important not to compare yourself to others. Physical activity doesn't always have to mean hitting the gym or following strict workout routines. Incorporating more movement into your daily life – like walking, stretching, dancing or taking the stairs – can make a big difference to how you feel. Moving regularly not only boosts physical health but also helps to reduce stress and improve mood, which will then feed into the nutrition decisions you make. My biggest tip is for you to incorporate more movement into your life without pressure or strict rules; consistency is key, and enjoying what you do will help you create those habits.

You don't need to be in the gym five times a week or run miles every day to reap the benefits of physical activity. One of my favourite exercises for my health is simply walking. I guarantee if you're able to increase your step count and take more regular walks throughout the day, it will change your life. It's low-impact, easy to fit into your routine, and highly beneficial for both mental and physical well-being.

## 5. CREATE A ROUTINE THAT WORKS FOR YOU

We often talk about consistency with diet, but routine in other areas of life is just as important. Try to establish a daily rhythm that includes regular meals, movement and time for self-care. It's about finding balance in all areas of life, not just food. By creating habits that support your health, you make it easier to maintain a positive relationship with both your mind and body.

'One of my favourite exercises for my health is simply walking. I guarantee if you're able to increase your step count and take more regular walks throughout the day, it will change your life'

# Daily Habits

## BREAKFAST HABITS: START YOUR MORNING RIGHT

1. I always say it's much easier to steal extra time at the start of the day rather than trying to claim it back later. Waking up a little earlier every day to curate a calm, productive morning sets you up for success, and taking just 30 minutes for a proper breakfast and a bit of movement can make all the difference in how the rest of your day unfolds.

2. The way you start your morning can shape your entire day, and building a strong morning routine will make it easier to maintain consistency in your diet and health goals. Begin with sunlight exposure: getting outside for just 10–15 minutes in the morning helps regulate the circadian rhythm that controls your sleep–wake cycle. Sunlight exposure first thing in the morning not only wakes you up more naturally but also improves your energy levels and mood throughout the day. If possible, combine your sunlight exposure with a morning walk. It doesn't need to be long – even a 10-minute walk can boost circulation, improve mental clarity and give you some valuable alone time to mentally prepare for the day ahead.

3. Preparing your breakfast the night before, or knowing *what* you are going to eat, can help eliminate any morning stress and ensure you start your day with a nourishing meal. Aim for breakfast options high in fibre and protein, which will keep you feeling full for longer, stabilise your blood sugar and provide a sustained release of energy. Prepping ahead allows you to avoid rushing out of the house without properly fuelling yourself, leaving you starving by mid-morning and reaching for the sugary snacks.

## LUNCH HABITS

1. Staying consistent with healthy eating during the busy workday can be challenging, but it's all about building small, sustainable habits into your lunchtime routine. Start by prepping your lunch the night before or at the start of the week. This doesn't mean you need a full meal plan – just prepping some key ingredients like grains, proteins and roasted vegetables, or many of the prepable lunches in this book, will help you put together nutritious lunches that will keep you full and energised.

2. To avoid the notorious post-lunch slump, which often strikes around 2–3 p.m., consider incorporating light movement into your routine after eating. A quick 10–15 minute walk, or simply standing and stretching, can boost blood flow and reduce feelings of sluggishness. Movement after eating has been shown to help regulate blood sugar levels, reducing the likelihood of feeling tired or craving those sugary snacks later in the day. If you're stuck at your desk, set an alarm to remind yourself to get up and stretch regularly – this can help prevent stiffness, improve focus and keep your energy levels steady throughout the afternoon.

3. Finally, building a consistent lunchtime routine – whether you're in the office or working from home – helps you stay on track. Set a dedicated time for lunch, step away from work, and use this time to focus on refuelling both your body and your mind. Taking 30 minutes for a proper, balanced meal – without being distracted by laptops or phones – will make your afternoon more productive and help you avoid relying on quick, unhealthy options.

## SNACKING HABITS

1. Snacking is often seen as a negative habit, but when done mindfully it can actually be an important part of a balanced, healthy diet. It's important to recognise that snacking isn't 'bad'. In fact, regular, balanced snacks can prevent overeating later on and help you maintain stable energy throughout the day.

2. The key is to use snacking as a way to support your main meals rather than replacing them or filling gaps out of boredom. The first step is to plan your snacks: think of them as mini-meals that provide

'A great habit to develop is learning a few quick and healthy dinner recipes you can make in under 15 minutes for those days when you're short on time or energy' nourishment between breakfast, lunch and dinner. Ideally, snacks should be balanced, with protein, fibre and healthy fats to help keep you full and stabilise your energy levels.

3. Another great way to build healthy snacking habits is to prepare your snacks ahead of time (and there's lots of recipe inspiration in this book to help with this). Having nutritious options ready and available makes it easier to reach for something healthy. If you're working from home, portion out your snacks in advance so you're not tempted to graze mindlessly throughout the day.

## DINNER HABITS

1. Dinner is not only the time to nourish your body, but it's also an opportunity to start winding down for the evening. To build a strong dinnertime routine, aim to eat at least 2–3 hours before bed. Eating too close to bedtime can interfere with digestion and disrupt sleep. Your body needs time to break down your meal properly; finishing dinner a few hours earlier helps you avoid discomfort and promotes a better night's sleep.

2. Another great habit to develop is learning a few quick and healthy dinner recipes you can make in under 15 minutes for those days when you're short on time or energy. Keeping it simple is key here; having a few go-to recipes from this book up your sleeve means you're less likely to turn to takeaway or convenience foods.

3. After your meal, create a calming environment to prepare for a good night's sleep: dim the lights, reduce screen time and engage in relaxing activities like reading or journaling. Pop the kettle on to have a digestive tea, such as mint, ginger or fennel. A consistent evening routine can improve sleep quality and set you up for a successful start the next day.

# Breakfast

Cottage Cheese and Oat Protein Pancakes | *Breakfast Bruschetta* | Herby Fluffy Folded Eggs | *Apple Crumble Oat Pots* | Super Beans on Toast | *Smashed Breakfast Sausage Tacos* | Spiced Harissa Turkish Eggs | *Tiramisu-inspired Granola* | Balsamic Mushroom Stuffed Omelette | *Apple and Cinnamon Fibre Prepable Oat Mix* | Baked Spinach, Feta and Sun-dried Tomato Eggs | *Breakfast Lemon Blueberry Muffins* | Smashed Peas and Poached Eggs | *Olive Oil Honey Toasted Oats with Greek Yogurt and Strawberry Compote* | Super Greens Shakshuka | *Fluffy Cinnamon Protein French Toast* | Stuffed Breakfast Chicken Sausage Pittas | *Sweet Potato Fritters with Soft-boiled Six-minute Eggs and Dill Yogurt* | Smoked Salmon and Cream Cheese Sesame Flatbreads

*Soft, fluffy, slightly tangy and fudgy, these pancakes are incredibly addictive. They're simple to make and the mixture can be blended until smooth if you prefer not to have little chunks of cottage cheese. Top with nut butter, maple syrup and berries for a filling, balanced and delicious start to the day.*

# Cottage Cheese and Oat Protein Pancakes

**SERVES 1**

**Under 209kcal,**

**12g protein per serving**

**FOR THE PANCAKES**

2 heaped tablespoons cottage cheese (low fat or regular)

1 heaped tablespoon plain (all-purpose) flour

2 tablespoons rolled oats

1 teaspoon baking powder

1 medium free-range egg

Zest of ½ lemon

1 teaspoon sugar or sweetener of choice

**TO SERVE (OPTIONAL)**

Nut butter

Honey or maple syrup

Yogurt and berries

Combine the pancake ingredients in a blender and pulse until smooth, but don't over-blend. Let the mixture sit for 5 minutes to firm up.

Heat a nonstick frying pan over a low-medium heat and add a little butter or oil if needed. Spoon tablespoons of the mixture into the hot pan, to form small, equal-sized pancakes. Making them small helps with flipping.

Cook for 3 minutes, then flip and cook the other side for 2–3 minutes until they feel light and springy to the touch.

Pair with nut butter, honey or maple syrup, a dollop of yogurt and fresh berries for the perfect high-protein breakfast.

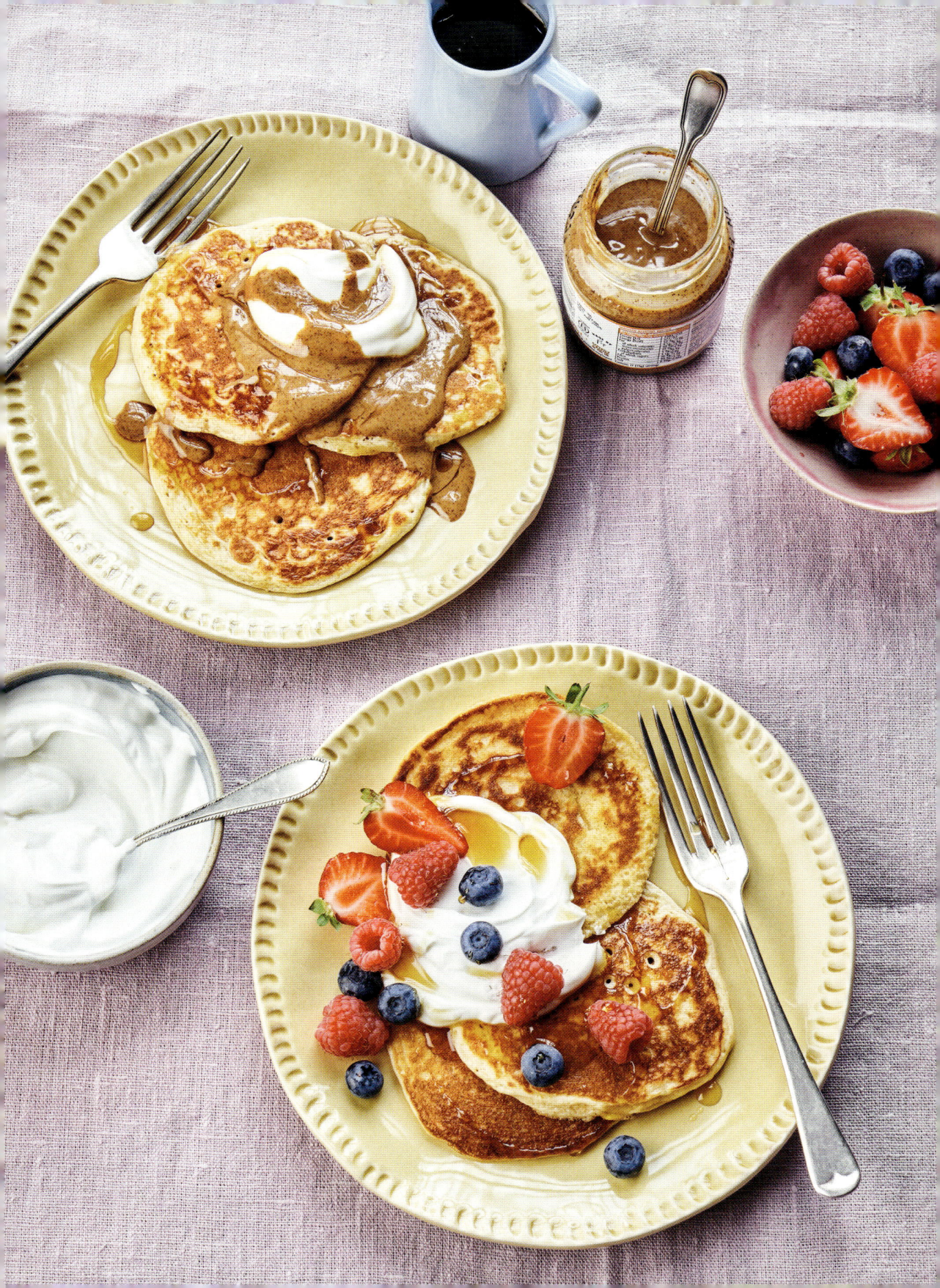

# Breakfast Bruschetta

**SERVES 1**
**Under 549kcal,**
**25g protein per serving**

2 medium free-range eggs

Large handful of cherry tomatoes, quartered

¼ red onion, finely diced

½ small ripe avocado, peeled and diced

Drizzle of olive oil

A few basil leaves

2 heaped tablespoons ricotta cheese

Zest of ½ lemon

15g (½oz) Parmesan cheese, grated

1 slice of bread, 40–50g (1½–1¾oz) – I like sourdough

1 small garlic clove, halved

Salt and pepper

Fill a small saucepan with water and bring it to a gentle boil. Add the eggs carefully and cook for 6 minutes for a soft-boiled egg, then place in a bowl of iced water to stop the cooking. Peel and set aside.

Meanwhile, in a small bowl, combine the cherry tomatoes, red onion and avocado. Add a pinch each of salt and pepper, plus a little drizzle of olive oil, then tear in the basil.

In another bowl, mix the ricotta with the lemon zest and Parmesan.

Toast the bread, then gently rub the cut side of the garlic clove over the surface of the bread 4 or 5 times, to add a subtle garlic flavour.

Spread the ricotta mixture evenly over the garlic-rubbed toast and top with the tomato and avocado mixture. Cut the soft-boiled eggs in half and place them on top of the assembled toast. Sprinkle with salt and pepper to taste.

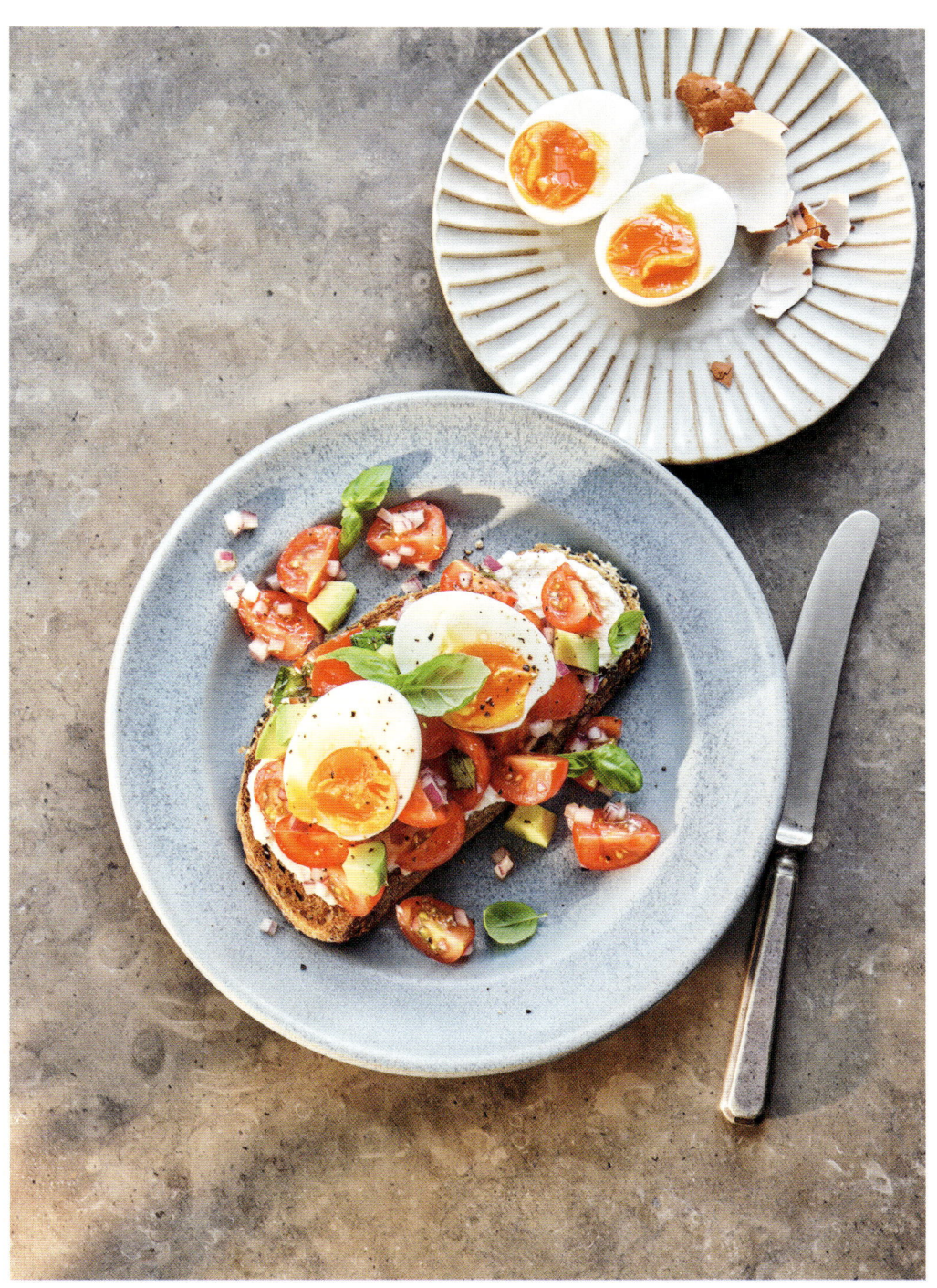

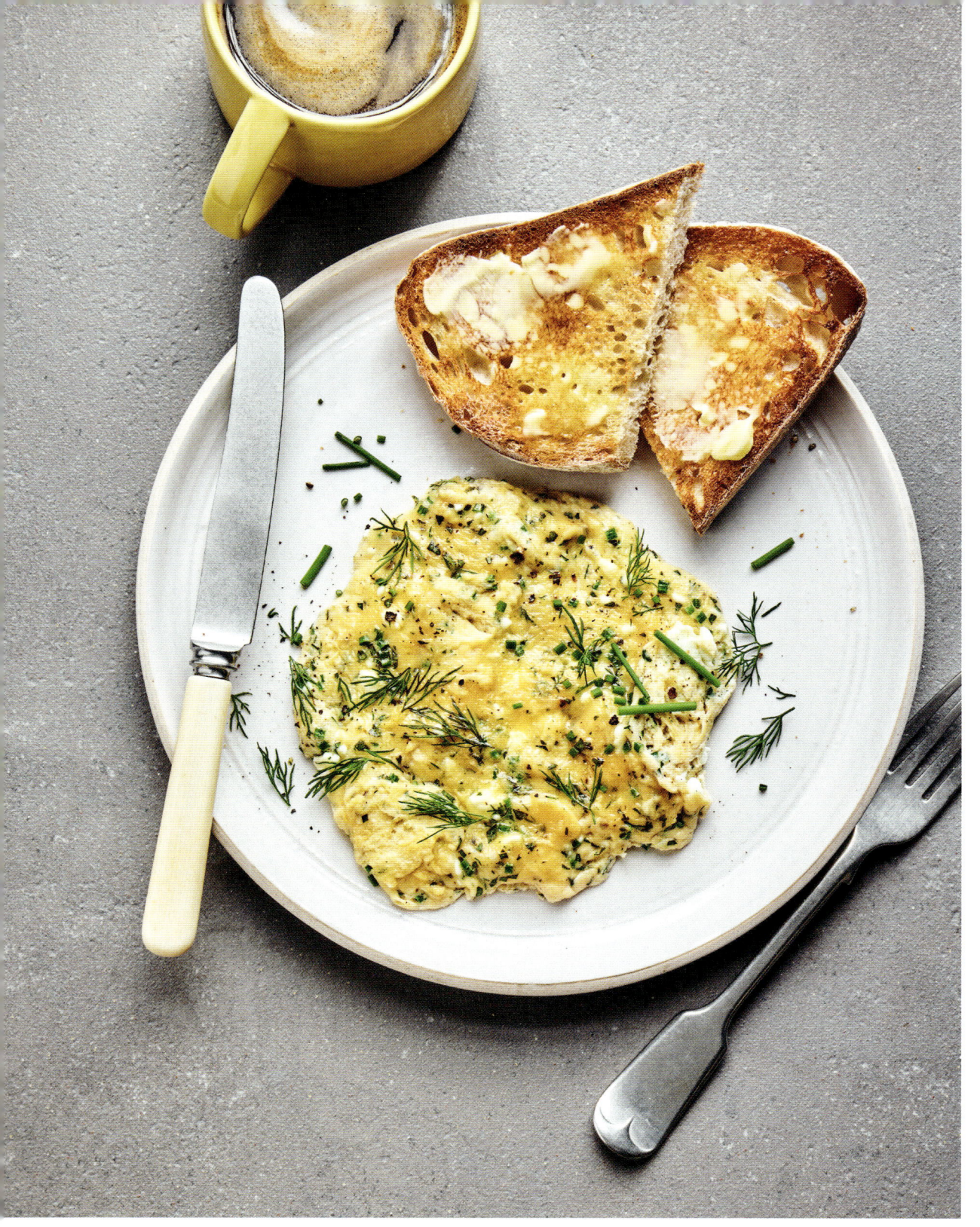

*Fluffy scrambled eggs with a hit of fresh herbs. This quick scramble is perfect for a light and nutritious breakfast packed with vitamins, antioxidants and anti-inflammatories to keep you full and energised.*

# Herby Fluffy Folded Eggs

**SERVES 1**
**Under 350kcal,**
**20g protein per serving**

2 large free-range eggs

1 tablespoon chopped
  basil, plus extra
  (optional) to serve

1 tablespoon chopped
  chives, plus extra
  (optional) to serve

1 tablespoon chopped
  dill, plus extra
  (optional) to serve

20g (¾oz) feta cheese,
  crumbled, plus extra
  (optional) to serve

1 teaspoon olive oil

2 tablespoons water

1 slice of bread, 40–50g
  (1½–1¾oz), toasted

Salt and pepper

Crack the eggs into a bowl and whisk them thoroughly. Add the chopped herbs and crumbled feta, season with a pinch each of salt and pepper and whisk again until everything is well combined.

Heat a nonstick frying pan over a medium-low heat and add the olive oil. Once the oil is hot, pour in the egg mixture. Let it sit for a few seconds without stirring, then gently stir with a spatula, pushing the eggs from the edges towards the centre.

As the eggs begin to set, pour the water around the edges of the pan and cover with a lid. This will create steam, helping to keep the eggs fluffy. Cook for another minute until the eggs are cooked but still soft and slightly runny.

Serve hot alongside or on the toasted bread. Sprinkle with additional herbs and/or feta if desired.

*This recipe combines the flavours of apple crumble but incorporates lots of healthy protein- and fibre-rich ingredients to keep things balanced. Topped with an almond and oat crumble, this is perfect for a make-ahead breakfast that can be batch cooked.*

# Apple Crumble Oat Pots

**SERVES 2**
**Under 461kcal,**
**16g protein per serving**

80g (⅔ cup) jumbo oats

200g (scant 1 cup) thick strained-style yogurt (Greek or Skyr)

1 large apple, grated (with skin)

1 tablespoon chia seeds

1 teaspoon ground cinnamon

1 tablespoon honey or maple syrup, or to taste

**FOR THE CRUMBLE TOP**

1 heaped tablespoon ground almonds

1 teaspoon jumbo oats, roughly blitzed

2 teaspoons butter, cold

½ teaspoon ground cinnamon

1 tablespoon brown sugar

½ teaspoon vanilla extract

Pinch of salt

In a bowl, combine the oats, yogurt, grated apple, chia seeds, cinnamon and honey or maple syrup. Mix well until all the ingredients are fully combined. Divide evenly between 2 jars or bowls.

For the crumble top, in a separate bowl, rub the ground almonds, oats, butter, cinnamon, sugar, vanilla extract and salt with your fingers until the mixture forms a crumbly texture.

Sprinkle 1 heaped teaspoon of the crumble top mixture evenly over each oat pot. You can store the oat pots in an airtight container in the refrigerator for up to three days.

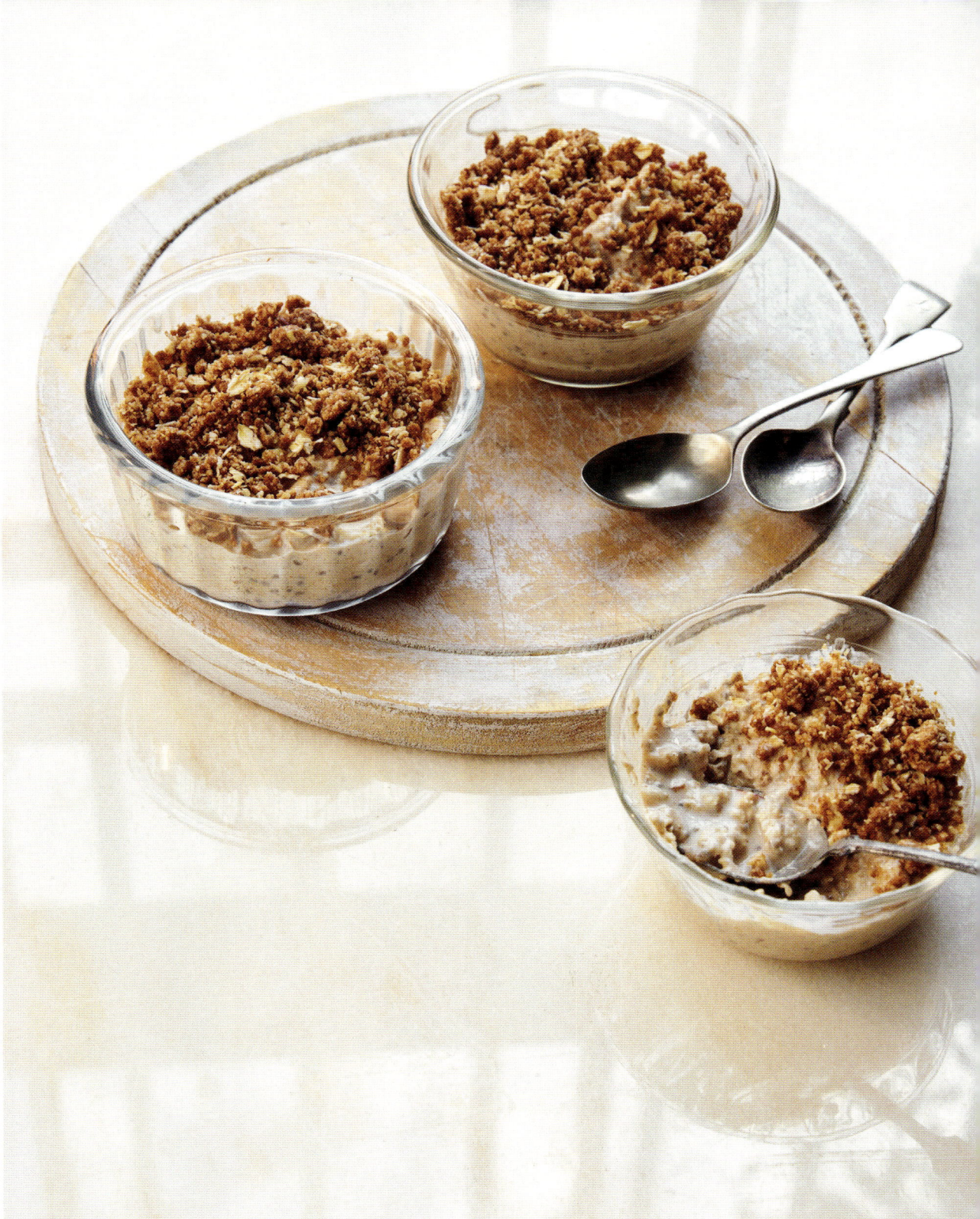

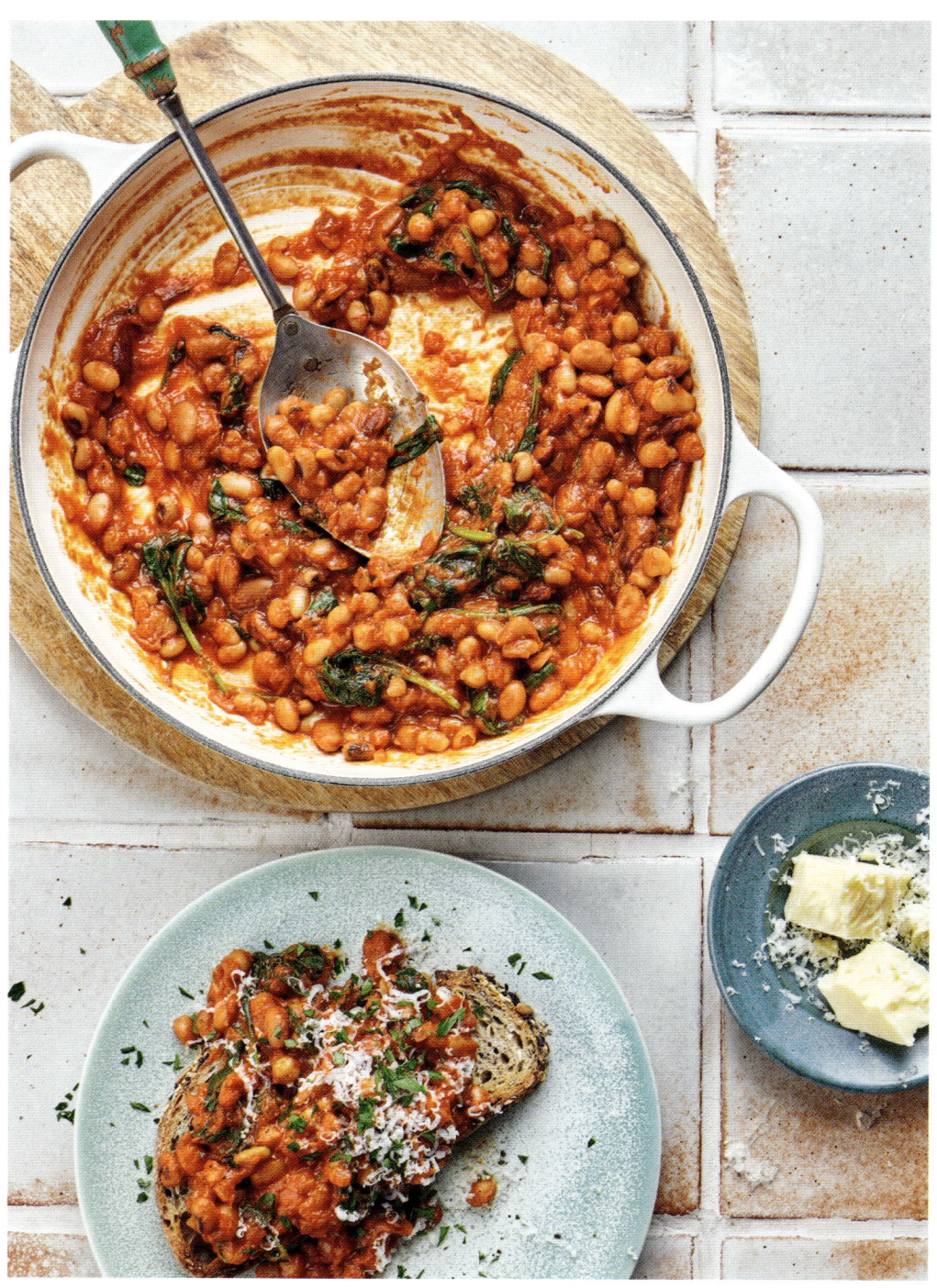

*Elevate the classic beans on toast with my homemade version, full of plant diversity and goodness. Did you know beans on toast is very nutritionally balanced, providing complete protein, lots of fibre and essential vitamins, making it a hearty and satisfying breakfast? Double or triple the recipe to batch cook; it's freezer-friendly, too.*

# Super Beans on Toast

**SERVES 4**
**Under 210kcal,**
**18g protein per serving**

300ml (1¼ cups) passata (puréed canned tomatoes)

2 roasted red (bell) peppers from a jar

2 teaspoons olive oil

½ red onion, finely diced

1 garlic clove, minced

1 teaspoon smoked paprika

¼ teaspoon dried chilli flakes (optional)

400g (14oz) can of mixed beans, drained and rinsed

1 tablespoon tomato purée (paste)

1 teaspoon Worcestershire sauce (optional)

Handful of baby spinach leaves

Salt and pepper

**TO SERVE (PER PERSON)**

1 slice of bread, toasted

15g (½oz) cheese of choice (I like a sharp Cheddar), grated

Chopped parsley, to garnish

In a blender, whizz together the passata and red peppers until combined.

Heat the oil in a large pan over a medium heat. Add the red onion and cook until softened, about 5 minutes. Add the garlic, smoked paprika and chilli flakes, if using, and cook for another 1–2 minutes until fragrant.

Add the mixed beans, tomato purée and passata red pepper mix to the pan and stir well to combine. Add the Worcestershire sauce, if using, and season with salt and pepper to taste. Bring the mixture to a simmer and cook for about 15 minutes, stirring occasionally, until it thickens (add a splash of water if the mixture becomes too reduced). Stir in the spinach to wilt.

Spoon the mixture generously over the toasted bread and top with cheese and some parsley.

*I love a breakfast taco, and these smashed sausage versions are a great easy breakfast or brunch that is always a crowd-pleaser. My version uses chicken sausages, but you can replace them with pork or vegetarian sausages.*

# Smashed Breakfast Sausage Tacos

**SERVES 2**

**Under 398kcal,**

**25g protein per serving**

8 chicken chipolata
    sausages, skinned

4 small corn or wheat
    tortilla wraps

Olive oil, for frying

Dried chilli flakes, to
    serve (optional)

1 lime, cut into wedges,
    to serve (optional)

**FOR THE SALSA**

½ medium ripe avocado,
    peeled, pitted and diced

2 medium tomatoes, diced

2 spring onions (scallions),
    finely chopped

1 teaspoon chopped herbs
    (parsley, coriander/
    cilantro or basil)

A few dashes of Tabasco
    (or to taste)

40g (1½oz) feta cheese,
    crumbled

Salt and pepper

In a bowl, combine the salsa ingredients, seasoning with salt and pepper to taste. Mix well and set aside.

Press 2 sausages gently on to each tortilla, using a fork or your fingers to spread them evenly to cover the surface. Heat a little olive oil in a large nonstick frying pan over a medium heat. Place the sausage-covered tortillas in the pan, sausage side down. Cook until the sausage is golden and cooked through, about 3–4 minutes. Flip and cook the other side for 1–2 minutes, until lightly toasted.

Remove the tacos from the pan and top with the salsa. Sprinkle with chilli flakes and place lime wedge on the side, if desired.

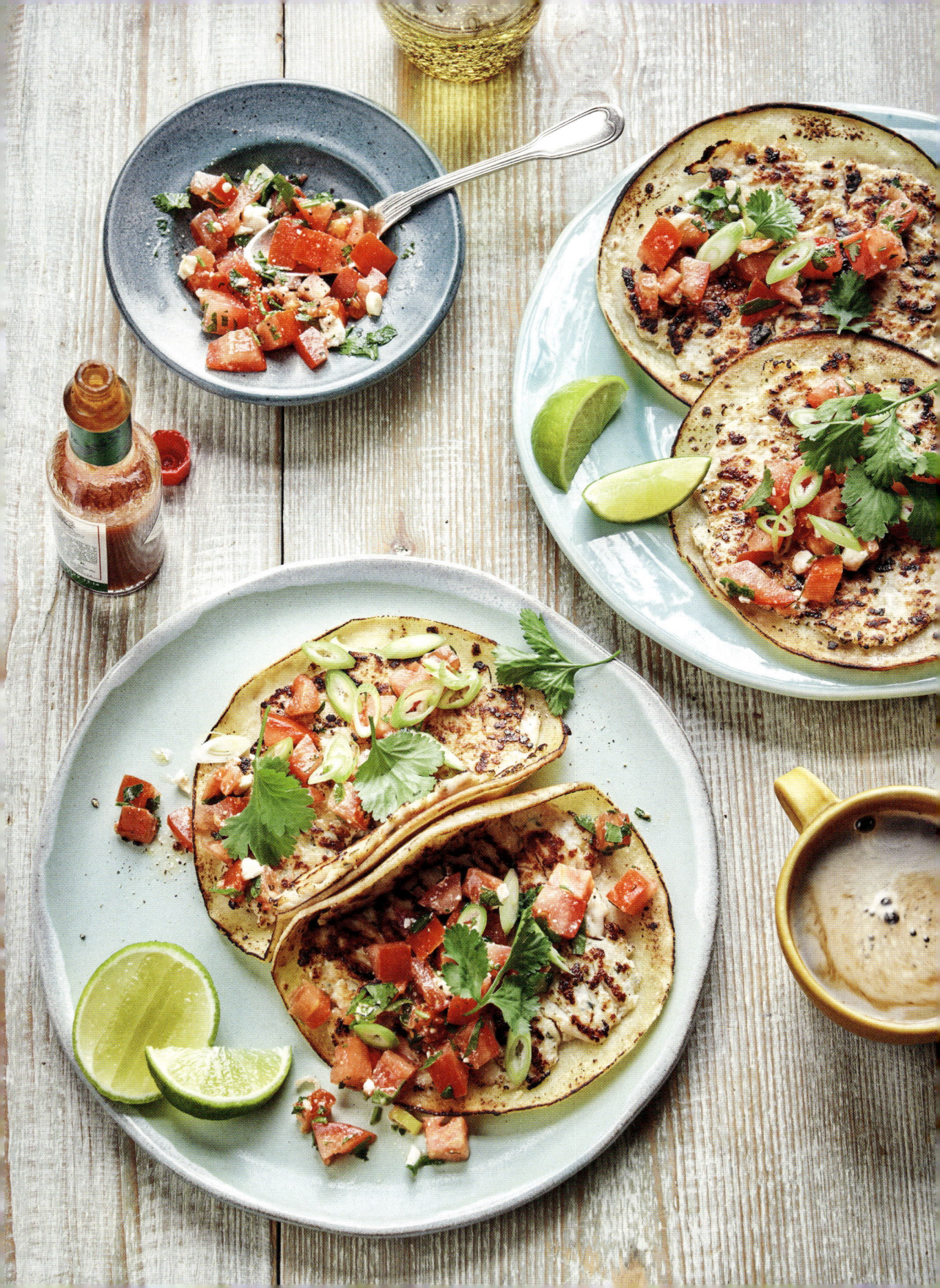

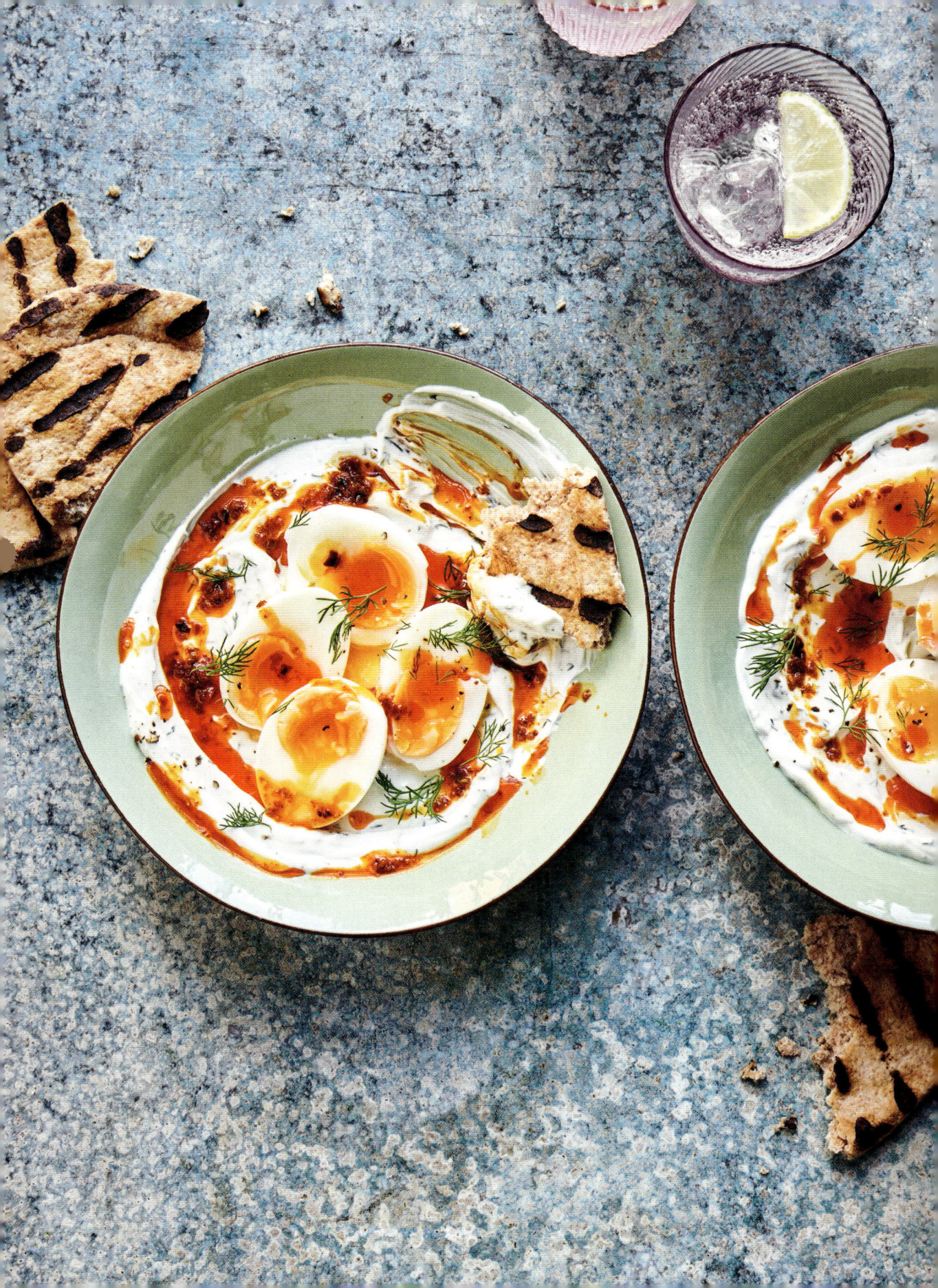

*Turkish eggs are one of my favourite breakfasts. I find it so much easier to get perfect eggs when boiling rather than poaching, guaranteeing oozy yolks and no watery whites. These eggs are served over a base of thick yogurt mixed with dill and garlic, and topped with a spiced butter.*

# Spiced Harissa Turkish Eggs

**SERVES 2**
**Under 417kcal,**
**30g protein per serving**

4 medium free-range eggs

200g (scant 1 cup) thick strained-style yogurt (Greek or Skyr)

2 tablespoons chopped dill, plus extra to serve

1 small garlic clove, finely grated

2 teaspoons salted butter

1 teaspoon extra virgin olive oil

1 teaspoon harissa paste

Pinch of dried chilli flakes

Salt and pepper

2 pitta breads, toasted, to serve

Bring a pan of water to the boil. Gently place the eggs in the water and cook for 6 minutes, then quickly plunge into a bowl of iced water and leave for 2 minutes. They should then peel easily.

Mix the yogurt with the dill, garlic and a pinch of salt. Taste and adjust the seasoning to your preference.

Add the butter, olive oil, harissa and chilli flakes to a saucepan, mix and heat until foamy and aromatic, then take off the heat.

Divide the yogurt mixture between 2 bowls, add 2 soft-boiled eggs to each bowl and drizzle over the spiced butter. Slice the eggs in half, finish with some extra dill, and add a pinch each of salt and pepper. Serve with warm toasted pitta for scooping and dipping.

*This combines the flavours of the classic dessert with the benefits of a nutritious breakfast. The granola is packed with fibre and is low in sugar; perfect for topping your favourite yogurt.*

# Tiramisu-inspired Granola

**MAKES 20 PORTIONS**
**Under 177kcal,**
**5g protein per serving**

100g (scant ½ cup) runny almond butter (or use cashew)

2 medium free-range egg whites

120ml (½ cup) maple syrup or honey

1 tablespoon instant coffee granules

1 tablespoon unsweetened cocoa powder

1 teaspoon vanilla extract

200g (2 cups) jumbo oats

100g (¾ cup) mixed seeds (e.g. pumpkin, sunflower)

150g (5¼oz) mixed nuts (e.g. hazelnuts, cashews)

100g (3½oz) dark chocolate, 70% cocoa solids, chopped into chunks

In a bowl, mix the almond butter, egg whites, maple syrup or honey, coffee granules, cocoa powder and vanilla extract together until smooth.

In a separate bowl, combine the oats, seeds and nuts, then combine with the almond butter mixture until everything is well coated.

To cook in the air fryer, lay a sheet of nonstick baking paper in the air fryer basket. Using your hands, sprinkle the granola mixture in a single layer on to the baking paper, keeping some clusters. Air-fry in batches at 120°C (250°F) for 12–17 minutes, mixing occasionally until golden (it will crisp up as it cools).

Alternatively, to cook in the oven, preheat the oven to 150°C/130°C fan (300°F) Gas Mark 2. Lay a sheet of nonstick baking paper on a baking tray. Spread the granola mixture in a single layer on the lined tray and bake for 15–25 minutes, mixing occasionally until golden (it will crisp up as it cools).

Allow to cool before mixing through the chocolate chunks. Store in an airtight container for up to a month.

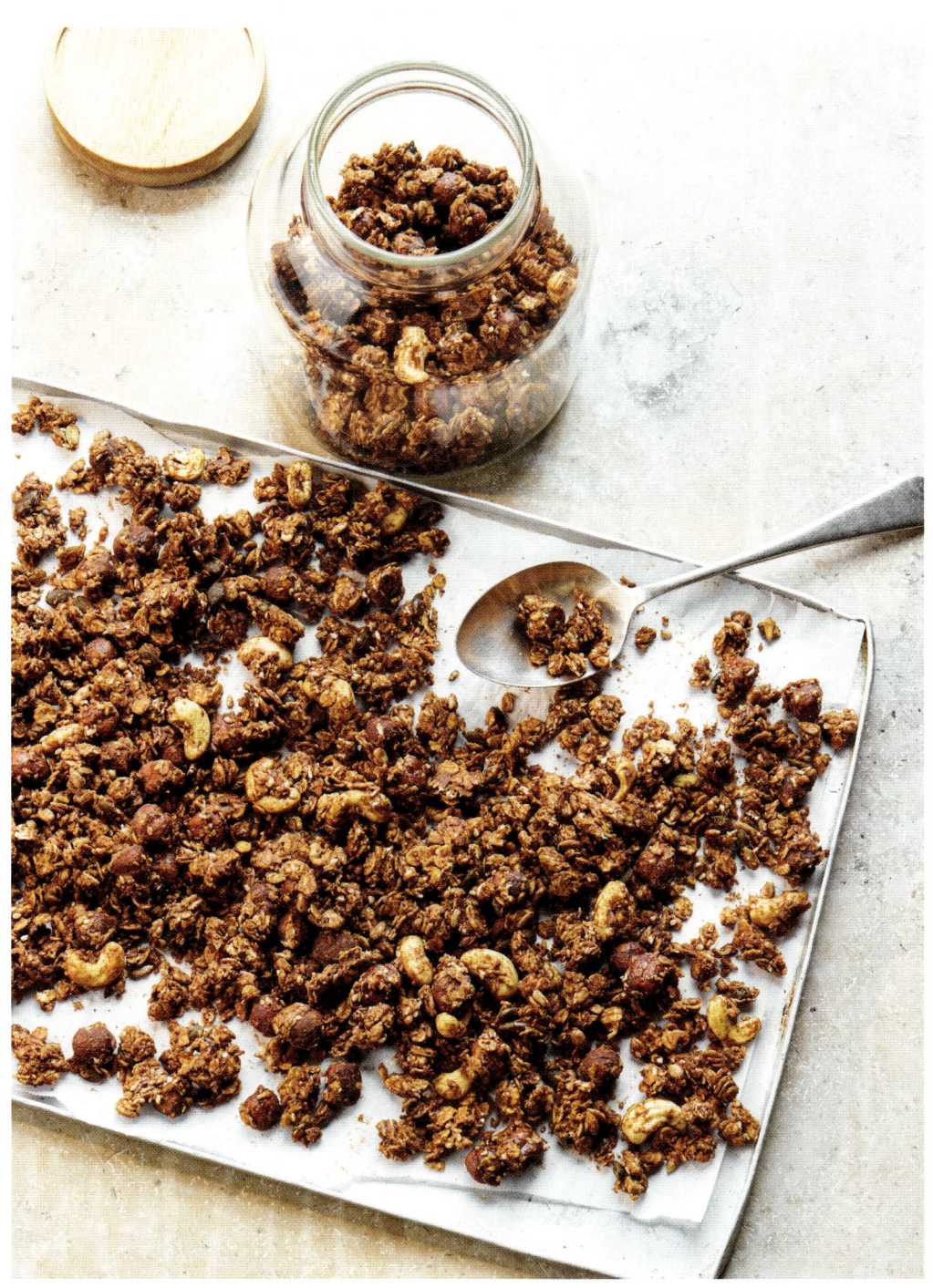

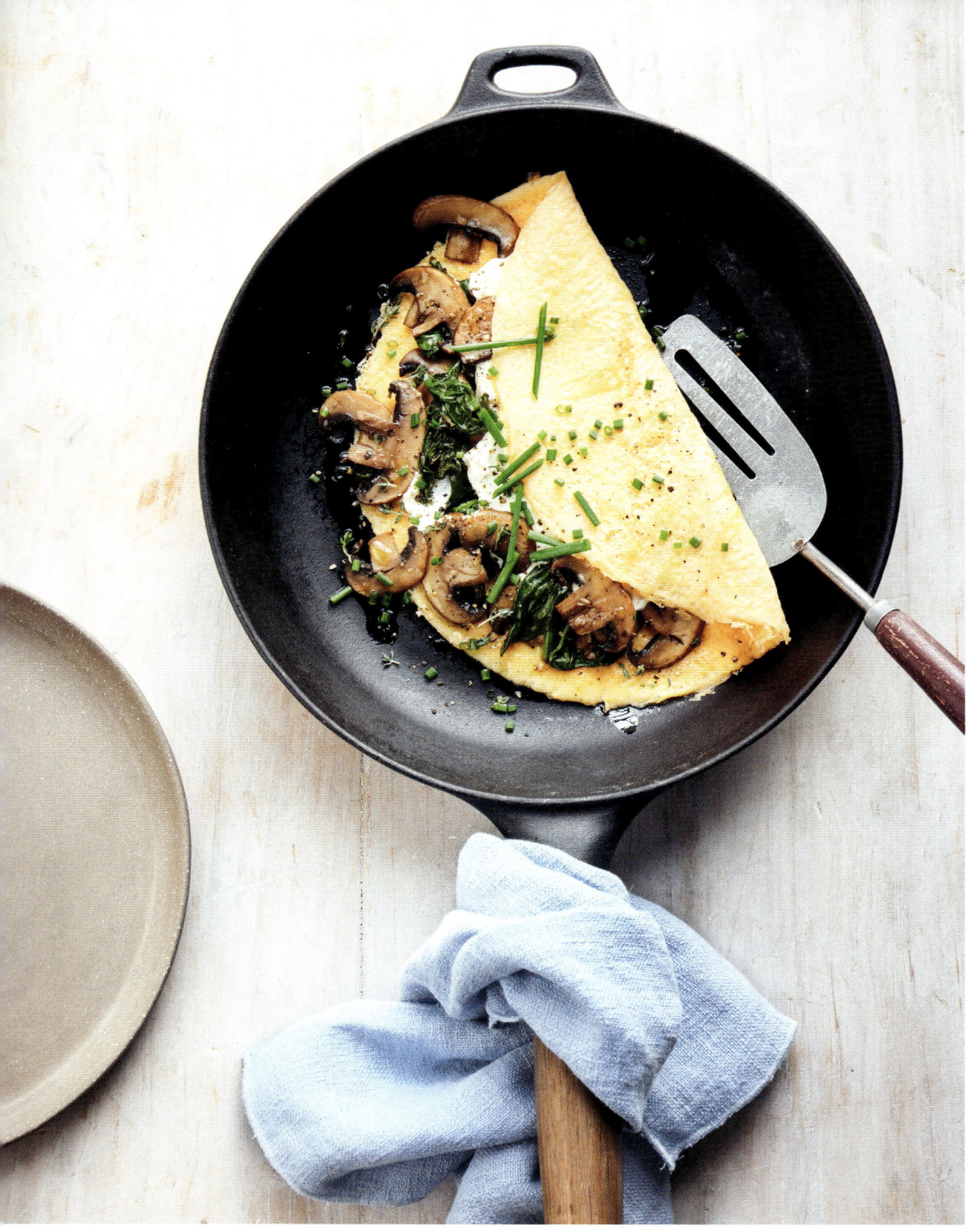

*I love a stuffed omelette. This one is made with chestnut mushrooms sautéed with balsamic vinegar and thyme and filled with cream cheese. Packed with protein and big flavour, it's perfect for a satisfying breakfast or brunch.*

# Balsamic Mushroom Stuffed Omelette

**SERVES 1**
**Under 275kcal,**
**17g protein per serving**

1 teaspoon olive oil

100g (3½oz) chestnut mushrooms, sliced

1 garlic clove, peeled

1 tablespoon balsamic vinegar

1 teaspoon thyme leaves, finely chopped

Handful of baby spinach leaves

2 large free-range eggs

3 scant teaspoons light cream cheese

1 teaspoon chopped chives

Salt and pepper

Heat the oil in a pan over a medium heat. Add the mushrooms and garlic clove and sauté until the mushrooms begin to soften, about 3–4 minutes. Add the vinegar and thyme and continue to cook for another 2–3 minutes until the mushrooms are fully cooked and the vinegar has reduced slightly. Add the spinach to wilt and season with salt and pepper to taste. Remove from the heat, remove the garlic and set aside.

In a bowl, whisk the eggs until well beaten, seasoning with a pinch each of salt and pepper. Heat a nonstick frying pan over a medium heat and pour in the beaten eggs, swirling to coat the bottom of the pan evenly.

Cook the eggs until they begin to set but are still slightly runny on top, about 2–3 minutes. Spoon the mushroom mixture on to one half of the omelette, add dollops of cream cheese on top of the mushrooms and sprinkle over the chives.

Carefully fold the other half of the omelette over the filling and let it cook for another 1–2 minutes until the eggs are fully set and the cream cheese is slightly melted.

Slide on to a plate and serve immediately.

*Dry oat mixes are a fantastic way to save time in the mornings without sacrificing nutrition. Prep your oat mix in bulk and, when you're ready for breakfast, all you need to do is scoop out a portion, add liquid (like milk or water), and cook in a pan or microwave – or have as overnight oats! Balanced, high in fibre and quick to prepare, this oat mix will make your mornings stress-free.*

# Apple and Cinnamon Fibre Prepable Oat Mix

**MAKES 10 SERVINGS**
**Under 225 kcal,**
**6g protein per serving**

400g (4 cups) jumbo oats

75g (2⅔ oz) dried apple slices, cut into small pieces

50g (scant ½ cup) whole almonds, toasted and roughly chopped

60g (⅓ cup) raisins

50g (⅓ cup) mixed seeds (e.g. flax, chia, pumpkin, sunflower)

2 tablespoons ground cinnamon

1 teaspoon salt

2 tablespoons thick yogurt, to serve (optional)

Scoop of protein powder, to serve (optional)

In a bowl, combine the oats, dried apple, almonds, raisins, seeds, cinnamon and salt. Mix well. Transfer the dry mixture to an airtight container to store.

For breakfast, measure out 1 portion (about 60g/2¼oz) of the mix. Stir in 150ml (⅔ cup) milk or water and heat in a small saucepan or microwave until cooked. Top the oats with yogurt or mix in a scoop of protein powder, adjusting the liquid as needed.

For overnight oats, measure out 1 portion (60g/2¼oz) of the mix into a jar or bowl. Add 150ml (⅔ cup) milk or water, and stir in optional protein powder or yogurt. Cover and refrigerate overnight. In the morning, stir, loosening the mixture with more liquid if needed, and finish with your favourite toppings, such as a drizzle of nut butter or fresh apple slices.

*Sometimes you just want a breakfast that's easy, balanced and satisfying – and this recipe delivers. It's packed with protein and is deliciously filling. It's one of those recipes that tastes so good despite being so simple to throw together, and it has become a weekly staple for me.*

# Baked Spinach, Feta and Sun-dried Tomato Eggs

**SERVES 1**

**Under 253kcal,**

**19g protein per serving**

2 large handfuls of baby spinach leaves, roughly chopped

1 spring onion (scallion), finely chopped

1 tablespoon chopped dill (or substitute with basil/parsley)

2 sun-dried tomatoes, drained and roughly chopped

35g (1¼oz) feta cheese

2 medium free-range eggs

Salt and pepper

Toast, to serve (optional, not included in macros)

Few dashes of Tabasco, to serve (optional)

Preheat the oven 190°C/170°C fan (375°F) Gas Mark 5, or the air fryer to 190°C (375°F).

In an ovenproof ramekin, roughly mix the spinach, spring onion, dill and sun-dried tomatoes. Place the feta cheese in the centre of the mixture, and crack the eggs around the sides, gently shaking the ramekin to distribute the whites evenly. Season with salt and pepper.

Bake in the oven or air fryer for 5–6 minutes, or until the egg whites are just set.

Remove from the oven or air fryer, and mash everything together. If desired, spread onto toast and finish with a splash of Tabasco for a spicy kick. Enjoy!

*Cake for breakfast is always a yes, and these lemon and blueberry muffins are nutritionist-approved with lots of protein and fibre to keep you full and balanced. Soft, fluffy, and perfect for a quick snack or grab-and-go breakfast, these muffins will keep for a week in the refrigerator, and are freezer-friendly.*

# Breakfast Lemon Blueberry Muffins

**MAKES 12**
**Under 184kcal,**
**7g protein per serving**

300g (1¼ cups) full-fat cottage cheese
100g (½ cup) brown sugar
50g (½ cup) ground almonds
150g (1½ cups) jumbo oats
100g (¾ cup) wholewheat flour (or use plain/all-purpose)
1 teaspoon baking powder
1 scant teaspoon bicarbonate of soda (baking soda)
Zest and juice of 1 lemon
2 large free-range eggs, lightly beaten
50ml (3½ tablespoons) skimmed milk
100g (3½oz) fresh blueberries

Preheat the oven to 190°C/170°C fan (375°F) Gas Mark 5.

In a blender or food processor, combine the cottage cheese and brown sugar and blend until smooth.

Add the ground almonds, oats, flour, baking powder, bicarb and lemon zest to a bowl, and mix to combine. Add the cottage cheese mixture, the lemon juice, eggs and milk.

Fold together until combined, but don't over-mix. Fold in the blueberries and divide evenly between 12 cups of a nonstick muffin tray. Bake for 30 minutes until risen and golden brown.

Allow to cool for 15 minutes before eating. Sweeten with a drizzle of maple syrup or honey, a dollop of yogurt and some frozen berries, or take a couple on the go.

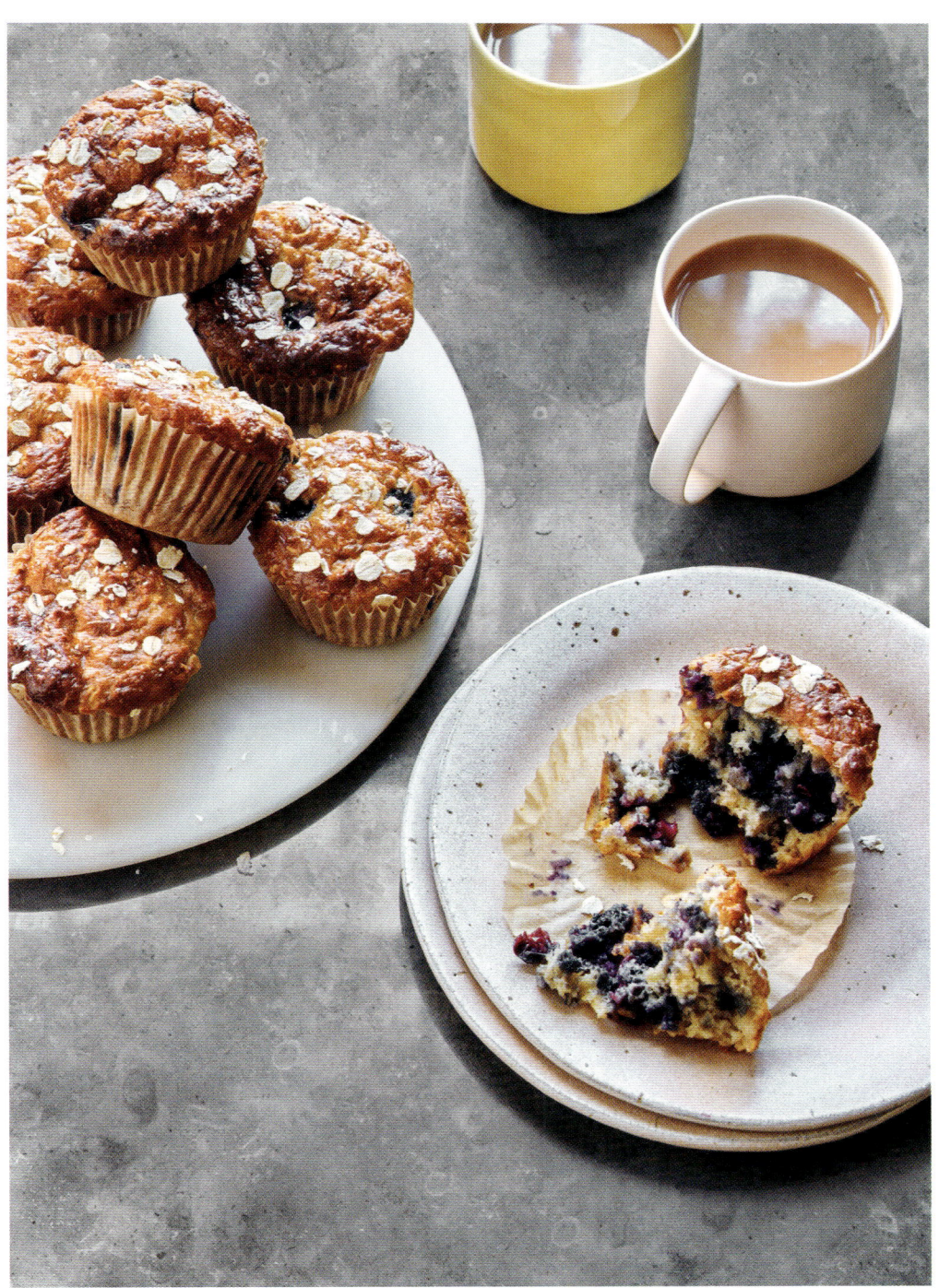

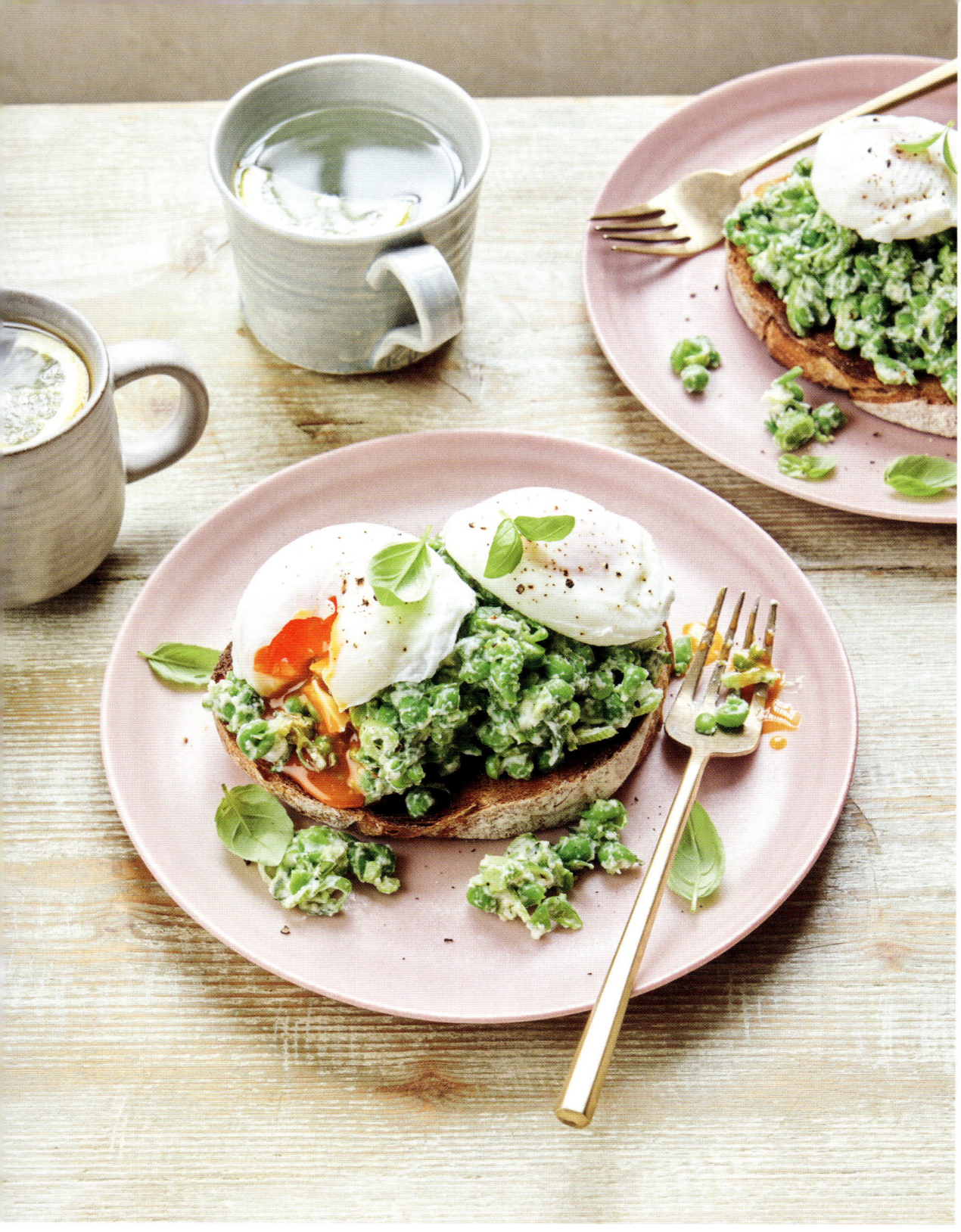

*This is a high-protein, nutritious breakfast that makes a lovely change from avocado toast. It uses the household staple of frozen peas, mixed with lemon zest, ricotta, Parmesan, basil and spring onions – topped with perfectly oozy eggs, the combination is so good. Keep the leftover pea mixture for a snack.*

# Smashed Peas and Poached Eggs

**SERVES 2**
**Under 410kcal,**
**29g protein per serving**

200g (1⅓ cups) frozen peas

50g (⅕ cup) ricotta cheese

30g (1oz) Parmesan cheese, grated

Zest of 1 lemon, plus a little juice

2 tablespoons chopped basil, plus extra (optional) to serve

2 spring onions (scallions), finely chopped

4 large free-range eggs

2 slices of bread

1 garlic clove, halved

Salt and pepper

Bring a pan of water to the boil. Add the frozen peas and cook for 3–4 minutes until tender, then drain and transfer to a mixing bowl.

Add the ricotta, Parmesan, lemon zest and juice, basil and spring onions to the peas and season with salt and pepper to taste. Use a fork or potato masher to gently crush the peas, mixing all the ingredients until well combined but still slightly chunky.

Fill a medium saucepan with water and bring to a gentle simmer. Crack each egg into a small bowl and gently slide them into the simmering water one at a time. Poach for 3–4 minutes until the whites are set but the yolks are still runny. Remove from the pan with a slotted spoon and set them on kitchen paper to drain.

Toast the bread, then gently rub the cut side of the garlic clove over each slice. Spread 2 tablespoons of the pea mixture over each slice and top with 2 poached eggs per person. Season with salt and pepper and garnish with extra basil, if desired.

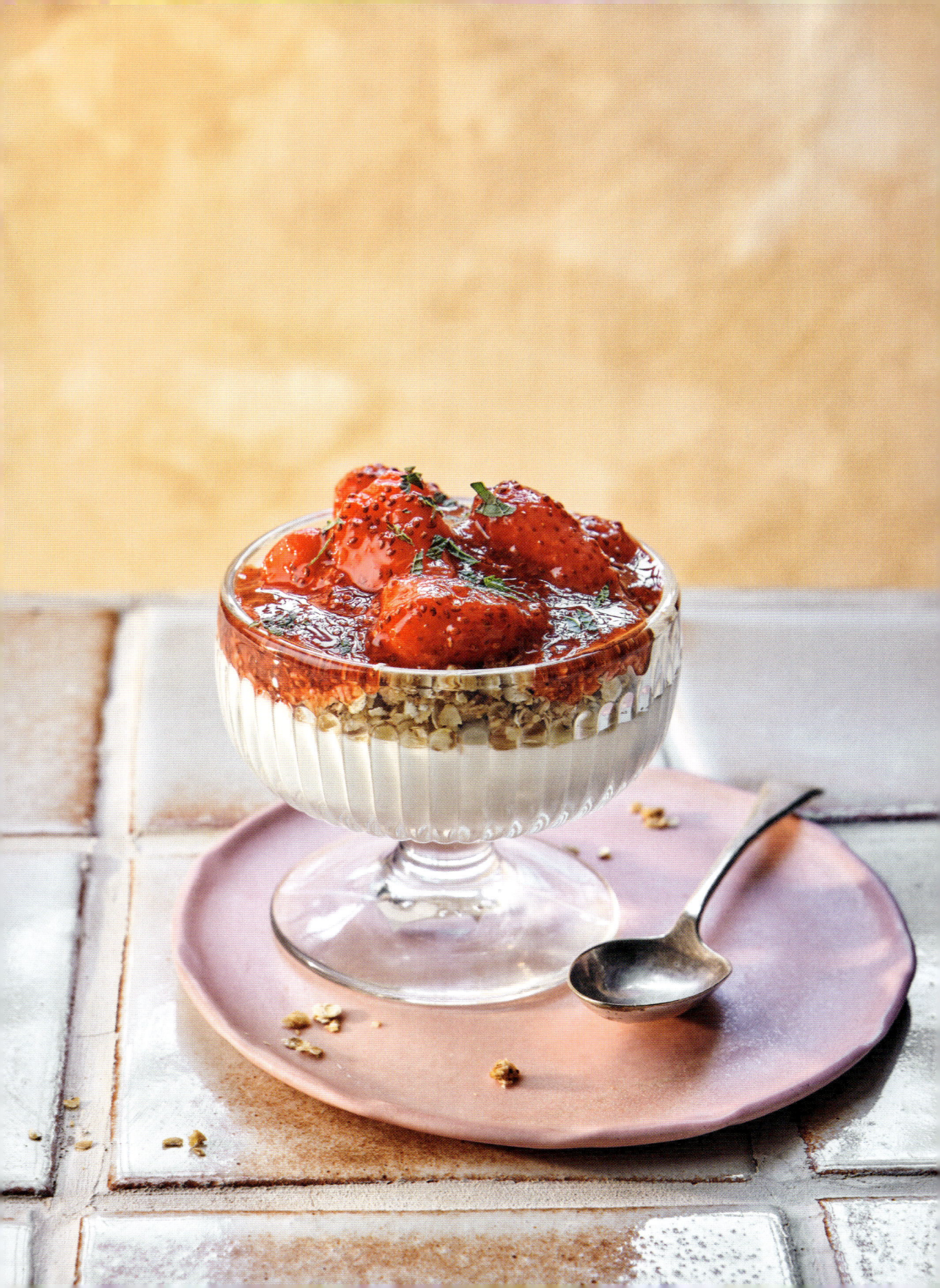

*A dreamy combination of thick yogurt, a three-ingredient granola
and high-fibre strawberry compote. I love to prep this and have
as a snack or something to settle my sweet tooth in the evening
because, as well as being balanced, it's absolutely delicious.*

# Olive Oil Honey Toasted Oats with Greek Yogurt and Strawberry Compote

**SERVES 2**

**Under 465kcal,**
**23g protein per serving**

1 tablespoon extra
virgin olive oil

2 tablespoons honey, plus
extra for the strawberries

Pinch of salt

100g (¾ cup) rolled oats

300g (10½oz) strawberries
(fresh or frozen), hulled
and chopped

1 tablespoon chia seeds

300g (1¼ cups) Greek yogurt
(or any yogurt of choice)

Chopped mint leaves,
to garnish

In a bowl, mix the olive oil with the honey and salt.

Add the oats to a large frying pan and lightly toast over a medium heat, stirring frequently, for about 4 minutes until golden. Drizzle in the olive oil mixture and stir to coat evenly. Continue to cook for another 4–5 minutes until the oats are well toasted, but watch they don't burn. Remove from the heat and let cool.

In a saucepan, cook the chopped strawberries over a medium heat until they start to break down and release their juices, about 5 minutes. Stir in the chia seeds and continue to cook for another 2–3 minutes until the mixture thickens into a compote. Remove from the heat and let cool, then sweeten to taste with honey (or use sugar).

To serve, divide the yogurt between 2 bowls. Top with the honey-toasted oats and a generous spoonful of strawberry compote. Garnish with mint.

*Note: You can store the toasted oats in an airtight container at room temperature for up to a week and the strawberry compote in the refrigerator for up to 5 days.*

*Absolutely jam-packed with green goodness and ready in under 15 minutes, this shakshuka is an amazing way to get in all of your gut-supporting greens without compromising on flavour. It's very versatile; you can use whatever greens you have in your refrigerator. Serve with toasted bread to dive into the oozing yolks.*

# Super Greens Shakshuka

**SERVES 2**
**Under 257kcal,**
**16g protein per serving**

Olive oil, for cooking
2 spring onions (scallions),
    finely chopped
2 garlic cloves, minced
1 tablespoon za'atar,
    plus extra to finish
2 handfuls of shredded
    kale or cavolo nero
8 pitted green olives, diced
150g (5½oz) frozen
    chopped spinach
150ml (⅔ cup) chicken stock
Zest of 1 lemon
4 medium free-range eggs
Salt and pepper

**TO SERVE (NOT INCLUDED
IN MACROS)**
Crumbled feta cheese
Chopped parsley
Dried chilli flakes (optional)
Toasted bread (I like pitta)

Preheat the grill (broiler) to medium.

Heat a little olive oil in a deep frying pan over a medium heat. Add the spring onions and garlic and sweat for 3 minutes until softened. Add the za'atar, kale or cavolo nero, olives and spinach. Sauté for 5 minutes, then tip in the stock and season with salt and pepper. Bring to a simmer and allow half of the stock to evaporate. Add the lemon zest and season with salt and pepper to taste.

Using the back of a spoon, make 4 little wells in the mixture for the eggs. Carefully crack an egg into each and cook for 2 minutes to set the bottom, then put under the grill until the egg whites are just set. The eggs will continue cooking in the residual heat, so remove them when still slightly wobbly to avoid overcooking the yolk.

Season the yolks with salt, pepper and a pinch of za'atar. Sprinkle over some feta and chopped parsley, with some chilli flakes if you like, and serve immediately with toasted bread.

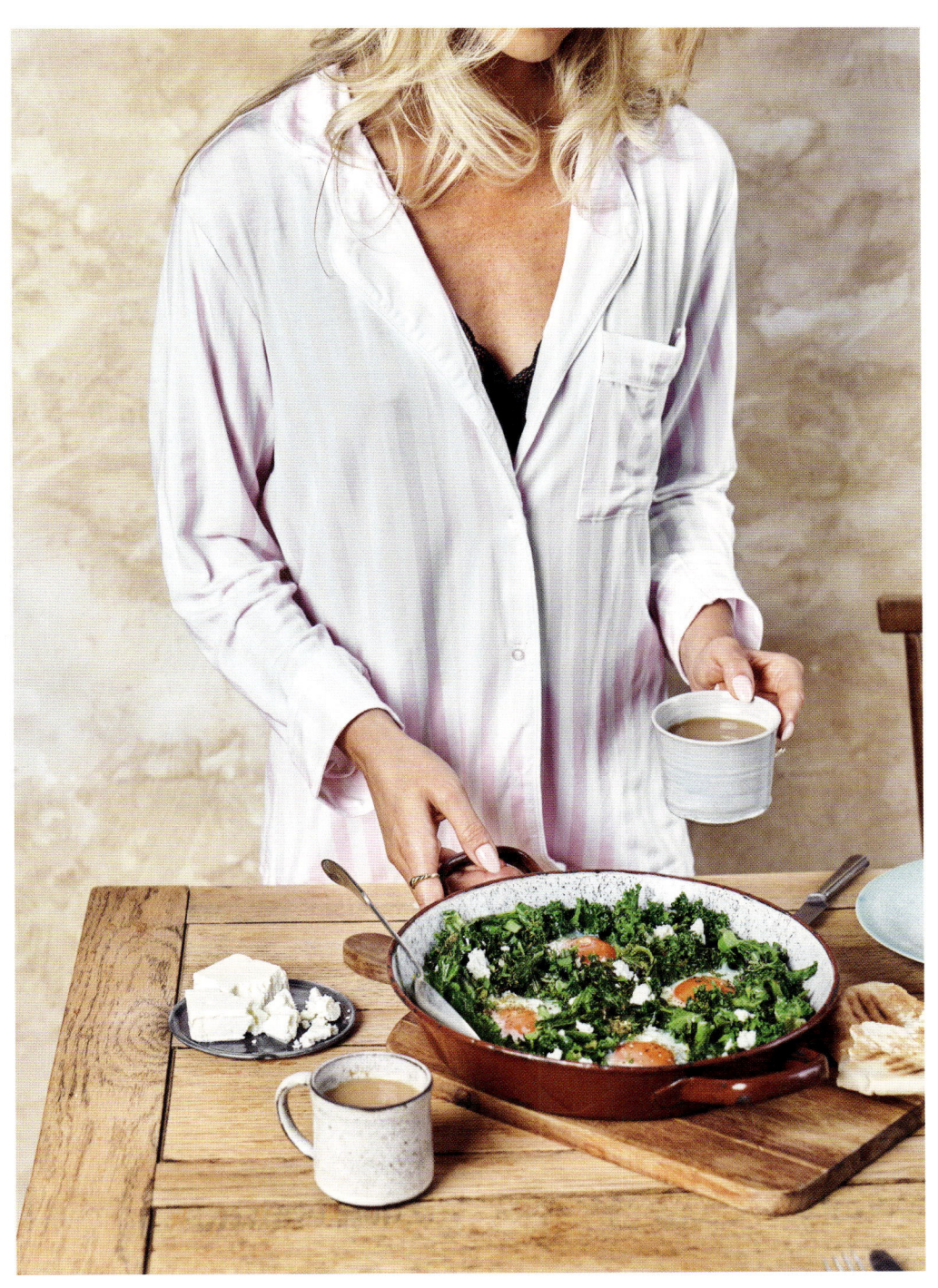

*This French toast is a healthier take on the classic, and perfect for a sweeter start to the day. It features an antioxidant-rich blueberry chia compote and a protein-boosted custard mix. High in fibre, protein and nutrients, this dish will keep you balanced, energised and ready for the day. It has a gorgeous custard-like texture on the inside and a crispy outside, perfect topped with yogurt and blueberry chia compote.*

# Fluffy Cinnamon Protein French Toast

**SERVES 1**
**Under 345kcal,**
**32g protein per serving**

1 large free-range egg, plus 1 egg white

60ml (¼ cup) semi-skimmed milk

½ teaspoon ground cinnamon

1 teaspoon honey, or sugar of choice

½ teaspoon vanilla extract (optional)

1 slice of bread (seeded or wholegrain)

Butter or oil, for cooking (optional)

**FOR THE BLUEBERRY CHIA COMPOTE**

500g (1lb 2oz) frozen blueberries

1 tablespoon chia seeds

**TO SERVE**

Generous dollop of yogurt

1 teaspoon nut butter of choice

For the compote, cook the frozen blueberries in a saucepan over a medium heat until they release their juices, about 5 minutes. Stir in the chia seeds and cook for another 2–3 minutes until the mixture thickens. Sweeten to taste with honey, or a sugar of your choice. Let cool.

In a shallow bowl, whisk together the egg, egg white, milk, cinnamon, honey or sugar, and vanilla extract, if using. Dip the bread slice in the mixture, flip, leave for a minute, then flip again and leave for another minute to soak up all the liquid.

Heat a nonstick frying pan over a medium heat and add a little butter or oil if needed. Add the soaked bread and cook for 2–3 minutes on each side until golden brown.

To serve, place the French toast on a plate, top with 2 tablespoons of blueberry chia compote and a dollop of yogurt, and drizzle with nut butter. Enjoy warm.

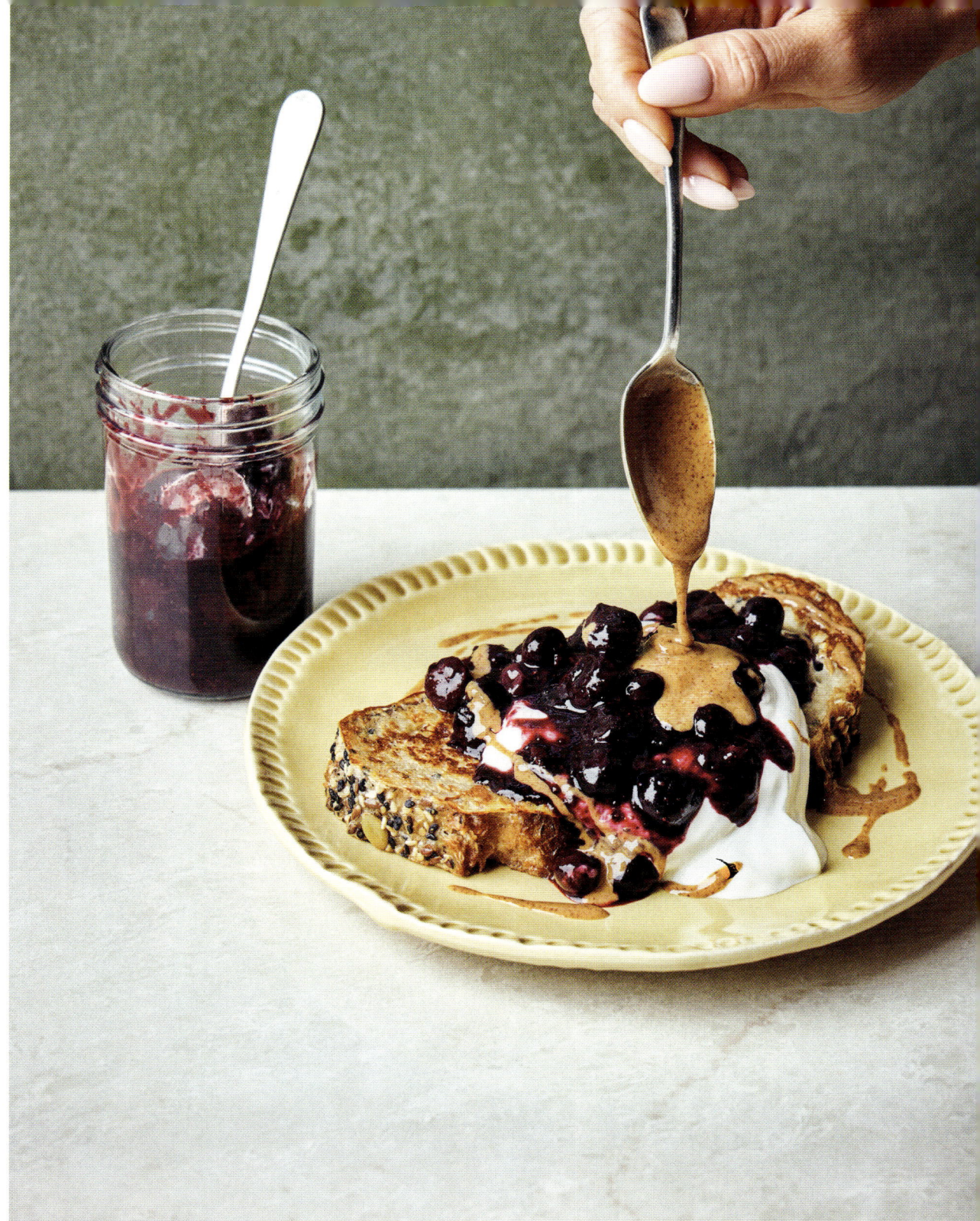

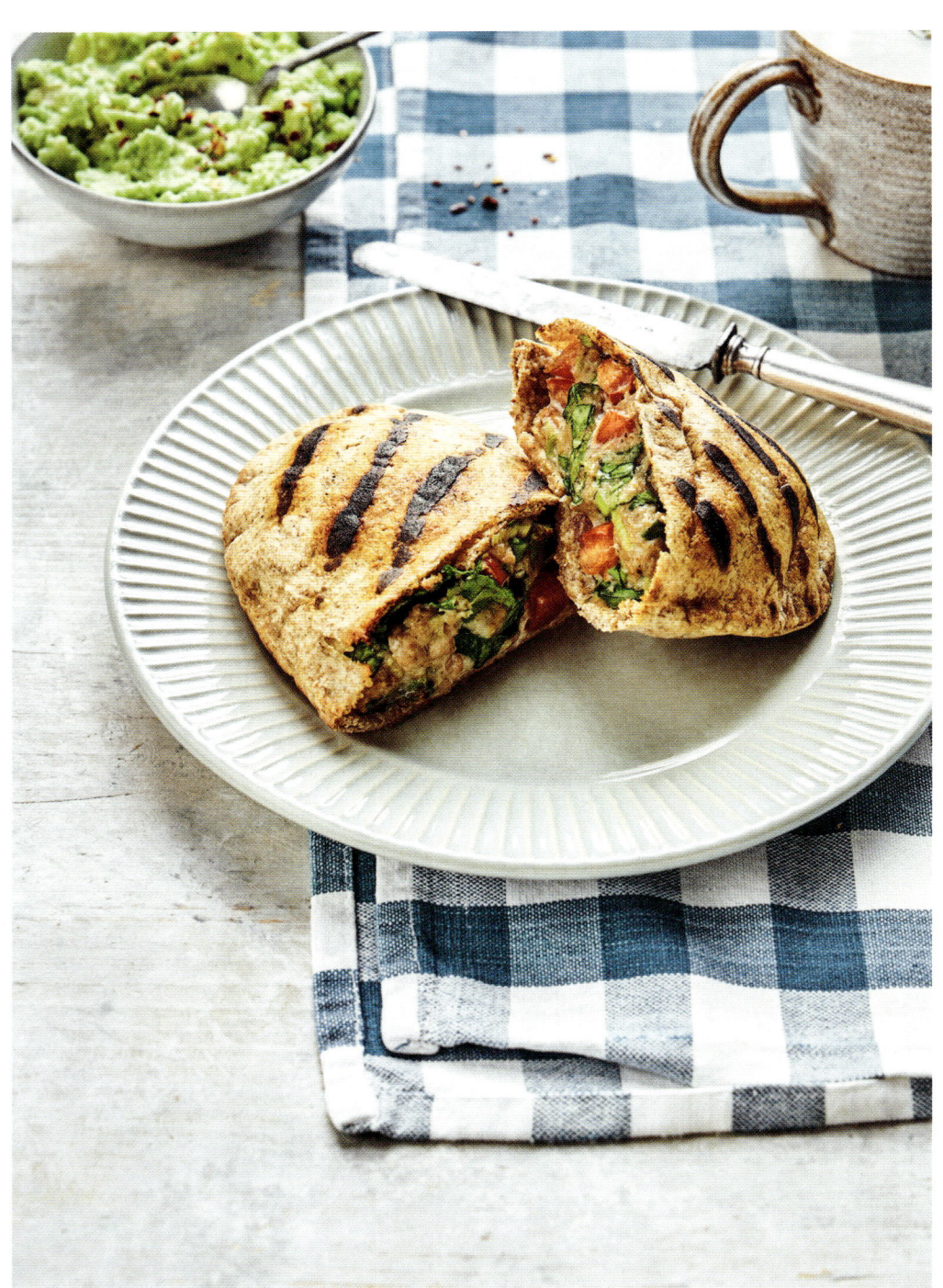

*Inspired by arayes, these stuffed breakfast chicken sausage pittas use high-protein chicken sausages to create a prepable, filling and balanced breakfast or lunch. Grill the pitta bread with the sausage mince and finish in the oven or air fryer if needed. Serve with creamy avocado for an ultra-satisfying meal.*

# Stuffed Breakfast Chicken Sausage Pittas

**SERVES 1**
**Under 282kcal,**
**24g protein per serving**

About 100g (3½oz) low-fat chicken sausage meat (or any sausage meat of choice)

1 medium tomato, deseeded and diced

Handful of baby spinach leaves, roughly chopped

1 large spring onion (scallion), finely chopped

1 tablespoon chopped basil or parsley

1 wholemeal (wholewheat) pitta bread

Salt and pepper

**TO SERVE (OPTIONAL, NOT INCLUDED IN MACROS)**
¼ ripe avocado
Juice of ½ lemon
½ teaspoon honey
Pinch of dried chilli flakes

Preheat the oven to 190°C/170°C fan (375°F) Gas Mark 5 (unless using an air fryer).

In a bowl, mix the sausage meat with the tomato, spinach, spring onion and basil or parsley, and season with a little salt and pepper.

Carefully cut the pitta in half across the middle to create 2 pockets. If you struggle to open them into pockets, microwave for 10–20 seconds to soften, then insert a butter knife or use scissors to open. Stuff each pocket with the sausage filling, making sure to evenly distribute it, and press it to the pitta so it's around 1cm (½ inch) thick.

Heat a griddle pan over a medium heat. Place the stuffed pitta in the pan and cook for about 3–4 minutes on each side. Transfer to the oven (or an air fryer at 170°C/340°F) and cook for 7–10 minutes, until golden and cooked all the way through.

Meanwhile, mash the avocado in a small bowl. Add the lemon juice, honey, chilli flakes and a pinch each of salt and pepper.

Remove the pittas from the oven or air fryer and let them cool slightly. Serve immediately with the mashed avocado, or prep to warm up later (see Note below).

*Note: These pittas are prepable and freezer-friendly. Once cooked, wrap them individually and store in the freezer for up to 3 months. Allow to fully defrost before reheating.*

*These fritters are perfect for brunch or even lunch. This recipe is so easy to double to make for larger groups, and the fritters are also freezer-friendly, so feel free to make them in bigger batches to turn to in the week.*

# Sweet Potato Fritters with Soft-boiled Six-minute Eggs and Dill Yogurt

**SERVES 2**
**Under 359kcal,**
**30g protein per serving**

2 medium-sized sweet potatoes, skin on, grated

2 large spring onions (scallions), finely chopped

5 medium free-range eggs, 1 beaten

2 tablespoons cornflour (cornstarch)

Olive oil, for frying

Salt and pepper

Lemon wedges, to serve

**FOR THE DILL YOGURT**

200g (scant 1 cup) Greek yogurt (0% or full fat)

2 tablespoons chopped dill, plus extra (optional) to serve

Zest of 1 lemon

1 tablespoon lemon juice

Combine the sweet potatoes, spring onions, 1 beaten egg and cornflour in a large bowl, and season with salt and pepper. Mix until well combined.

Brush a little olive oil in a large frying pan over a medium heat. Scoop a heaped tablespoon of the sweet potato mixture into the pan and flatten it slightly to form a fritter. Repeat with the remaining mixture, cooking the fritters in batches to avoid overcrowding the pan.

Fry the fritters on each side for 3–4 minutes or until golden brown and crispy. Transfer to a plate lined with kitchen paper to drain any excess oil.

Meanwhile, bring a pan of water to the boil. Carefully add the remaining eggs and cook for exactly 6 minutes. Remove from the pan and place in a bowl of iced water to stop the cooking. Leave for 2 minutes, then peel.

In a small bowl, combine the yogurt, dill, lemon zest and juice with salt and pepper to taste, and mix until well combined.

Place a few sweet potato fritters on each plate. Cut the soft-boiled eggs in half and place them on top of the fritters. Drizzle with the dill yogurt and garnish with additional fresh dill and lemon wedges if desired.

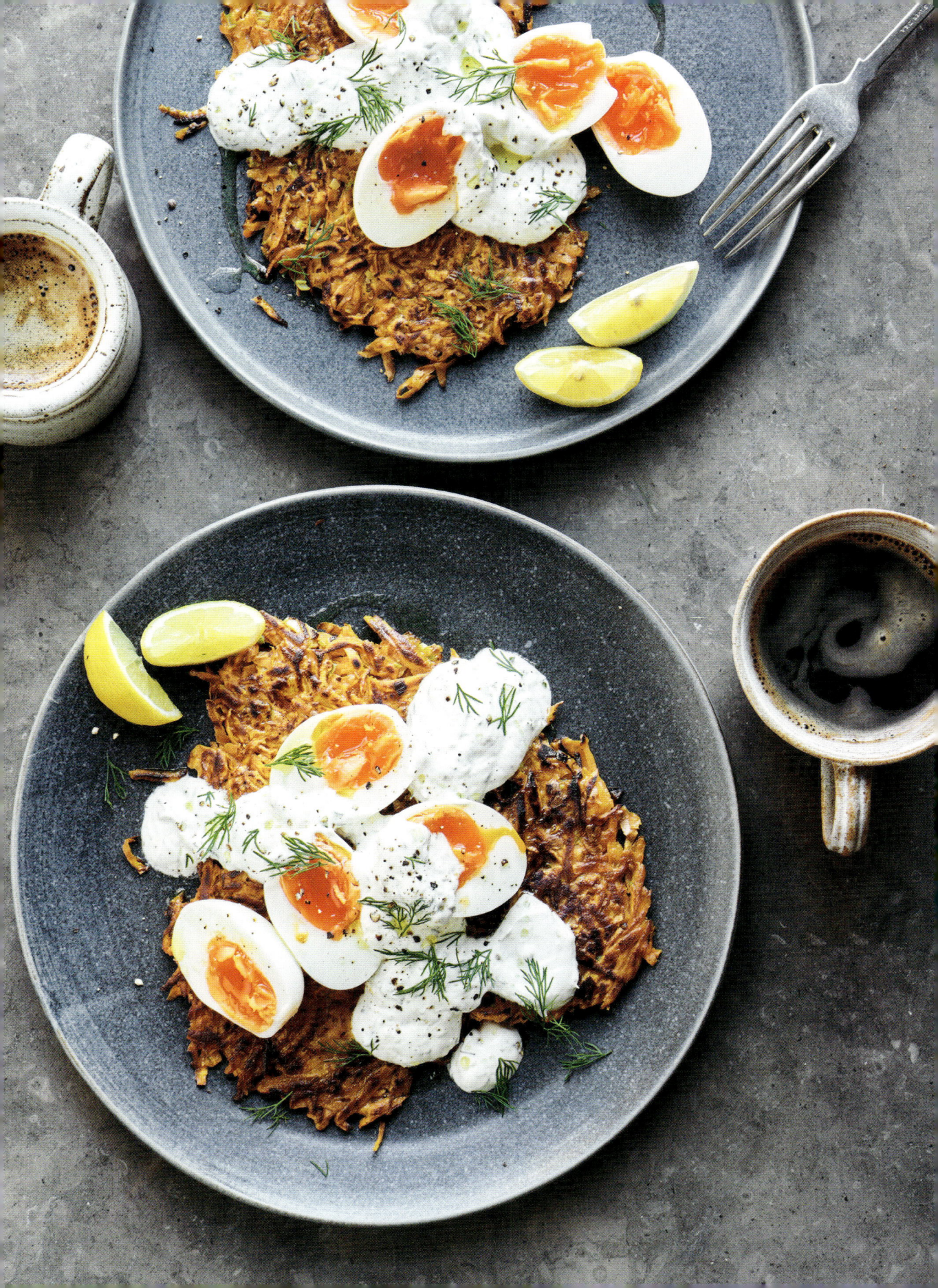

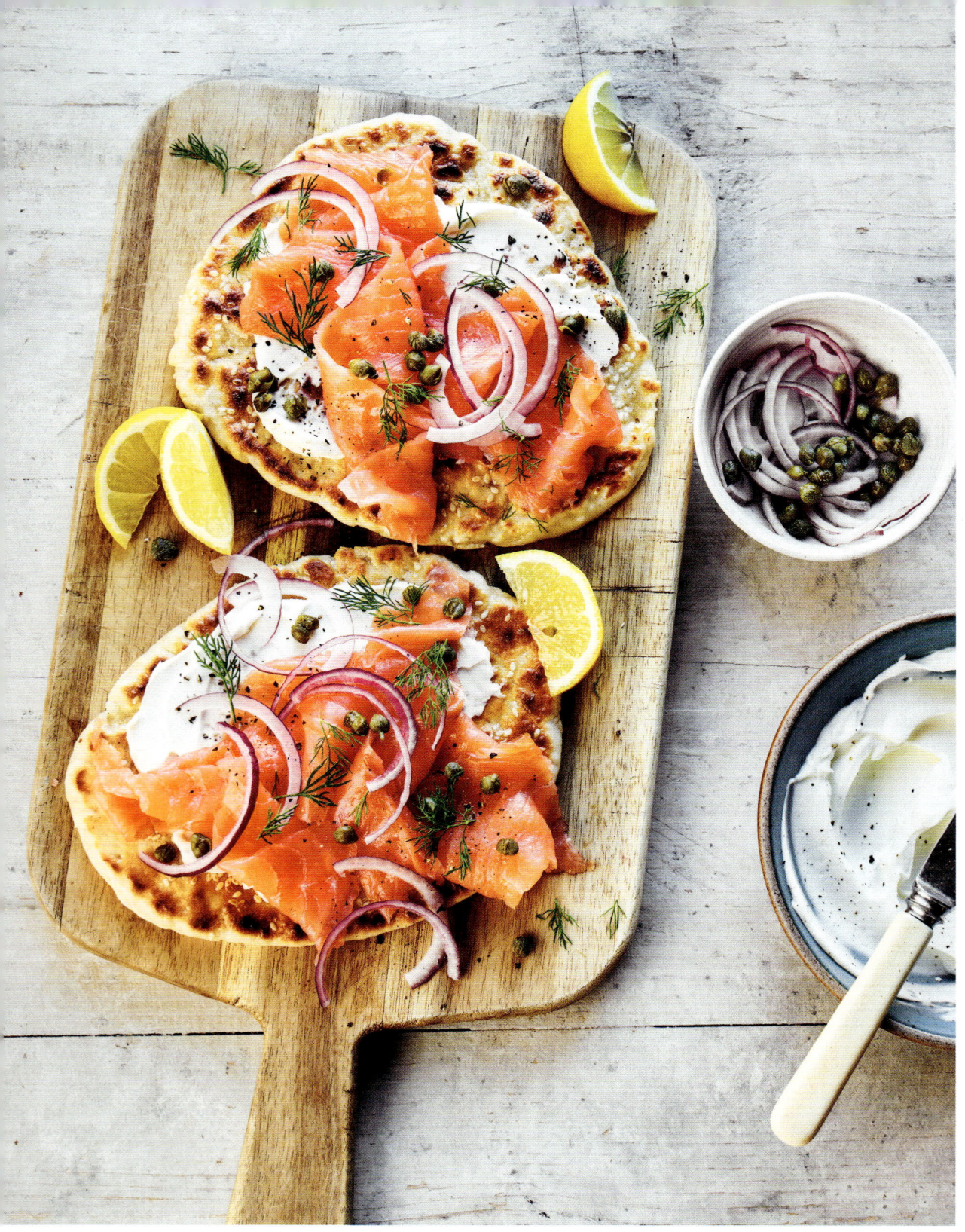

*All the flavours of my favourite bagel, but in a lighter homemade flatbread version. No need for endless kneading and resting; this dough uses just three ingredients and is ready in under 5 minutes. Stuff the warm flatbreads with rich smoked salmon, creamy cheese, tangy red onion and capers – perfect for a satisfying breakfast, brunch or light lunch. The flatbreads can be made in batches, and also frozen.*

# Smoked Salmon and Cream Cheese Sesame Flatbreads

**SERVES 2**
**Under 397kcal,**
**25g protein per serving**

2 tablespoons cream cheese
100g (3½oz) smoked salmon
¼ red onion, finely sliced
1 tablespoon capers, drained
Dill, to garnish (optional)
Lemon wedges, to serve

**FOR THE FLATBREADS**
120g (1 cup) plain (all-purpose) flour, plus extra for dusting
120g (½ cup) Greek yogurt (0% or full fat)
½ teaspoon baking powder
¼ teaspoon salt
1 tablespoon sesame seeds

In a bowl, mix the flour, yogurt, baking powder and salt together until a dough forms. Knead on a floured surface for a few minutes until smooth. Divide the dough into 2 equal portions. Roll each portion into a flat round, about 5mm (¼ inch) thick. Press the sesame seeds evenly into the surface of each round.

Heat a nonstick frying pan over a medium heat. Cook each flatbread on one side for 2–3 minutes until bubbles form and the bottom is golden brown. Watch the sesame seeds don't burn. Flip and cook for another 2–3 minutes on the other side.

Spread half of the cream cheese on one half of each flatbread. Layer the smoked salmon evenly over the cream cheese. Top with red onion and capers. Fold the flatbread over to enclose the filling.

If desired, cut each stuffed flatbread in half. Garnish with dill, if desired, and serve with lemon wedges on the side.

# Lunch

BLT Pasta Salad | *Halloumi Sweet Potato Jackets with Basil Yogurt* | Spicy Chicken Crunch Bagels | *Chopped Waldorf Salad* | Sticky Cashew Orange Slaw | *Super Greens and Feta Soup* | Creamy Broccoli and Basil Pasta | *Hot Smoked Salmon Potato Salad with Vinaigrette* | Tomato Tarts with Herby Feta and Ricotta | *Prawn Toast Toastie* | Salmon and Spinach Filo Cottage Cheese Quiche | *Crispy Smashed Potato Mackerel Salad* | Spinach, Goat's Cheese and Beetroot Tartine | *Protein Power Pea and Miso Soup with Whipped Ricotta* | Chicken Sweetcorn Egg Drop Soup | *Speedy Glow Wellness Bowls with Sticky Peanut Carrot Slaw* | Thai Red Coconut Gyoza Soup | *Crispy Baked Chicken Tacos* | Sesame Soy Noodle Salad with Shredded Chicken | *Crispy Baked Parmesan Chicken with Basil Goddess Salad* | Smashed Cucumber Greek Salad

*This makes a perfect lunch, using crispy Parma ham and a lighter yogurt dressing. It's ideal for prepping and won't go soggy when stored, and not only is it delicious, it's also super versatile – swap the chicken with any protein of your choice. Store refrigerated for up to 3 days.*

# BLT Pasta Salad

**SERVES 2**
**Under 427kcal,**
**32g protein per serving**

120g (4oz) dried pasta of choice (I like wholegrain rigatoni)

4 slices of Parma ham

160–200g (5¾–7oz) cooked chicken breast (or any protein of choice)

150g (5½oz) cherry tomatoes, halved

8 sun-dried tomatoes, drained and roughly chopped

1 little gem lettuce, leaves shredded

Salt and pepper

**FOR THE DRESSING**

3 heaped tablespoons Greek yogurt (0% or full fat)

1 tablespoon wholegrain mustard

Zest of 1 lemon and juice of ½

Small handful of basil leaves, chopped

2 spring onions (scallions), finely chopped

1 teaspoon honey

Bring a pan of salted water to the boil, add the pasta and cook according to the packet instructions. Drain into a colander or sieve (strainer) and leave to drip-dry.

Preheat the oven to 210°C/190°C fan (410°F) Gas Mark 6½, or the air fryer to 190°C (375°F). Place the Parma ham on a baking tray lined with nonstick baking paper and bake for 10–12 minutes, or line the air fryer basket with nonstick baking paper and air fry for 6 minutes, until crispy. Let cool, then break into pieces.

For the dressing, in a bowl, mix the yogurt, mustard, lemon zest and juice, basil and spring onions. Stir in the honey to combine, and add salt and pepper to taste; you want it punchy with flavour.

If using cooked chicken, shred it into bite-sized pieces. If using other proteins, like prawns (shrimp) or salmon, prepare them as desired. Set aside.

In a large bowl, combine the cooled pasta, cherry tomatoes, sun-dried tomatoes, lettuce and chicken or other protein. Add the crispy Parma ham pieces. Pour the dressing over the salad and toss to coat everything evenly.

*Note: To keep the salad from drying out, add extra dressing just before serving, especially if you are taking it to the office. If not serving immediately, store the salad in an airtight container in the refrigerator, to retain moisture.*

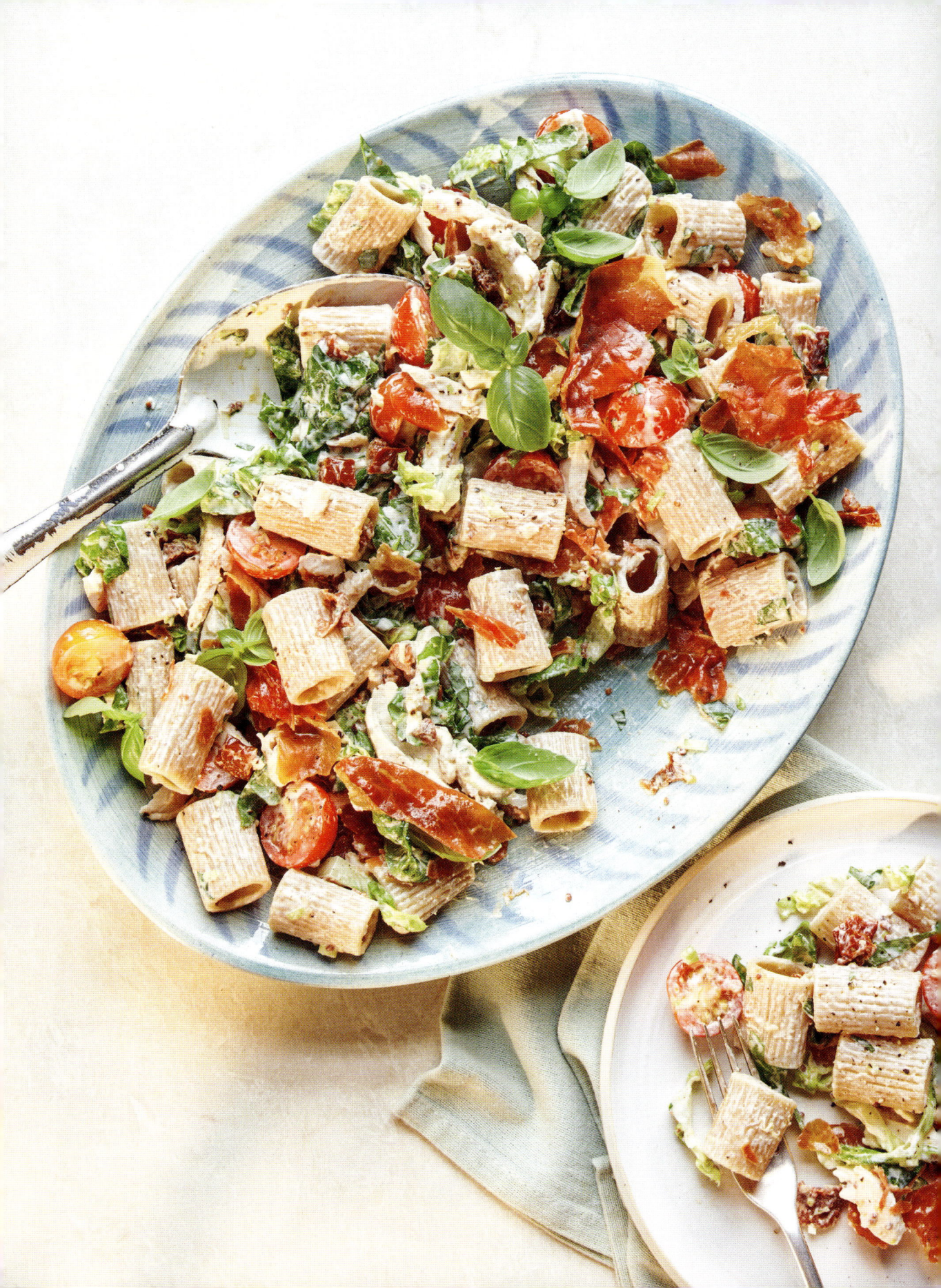

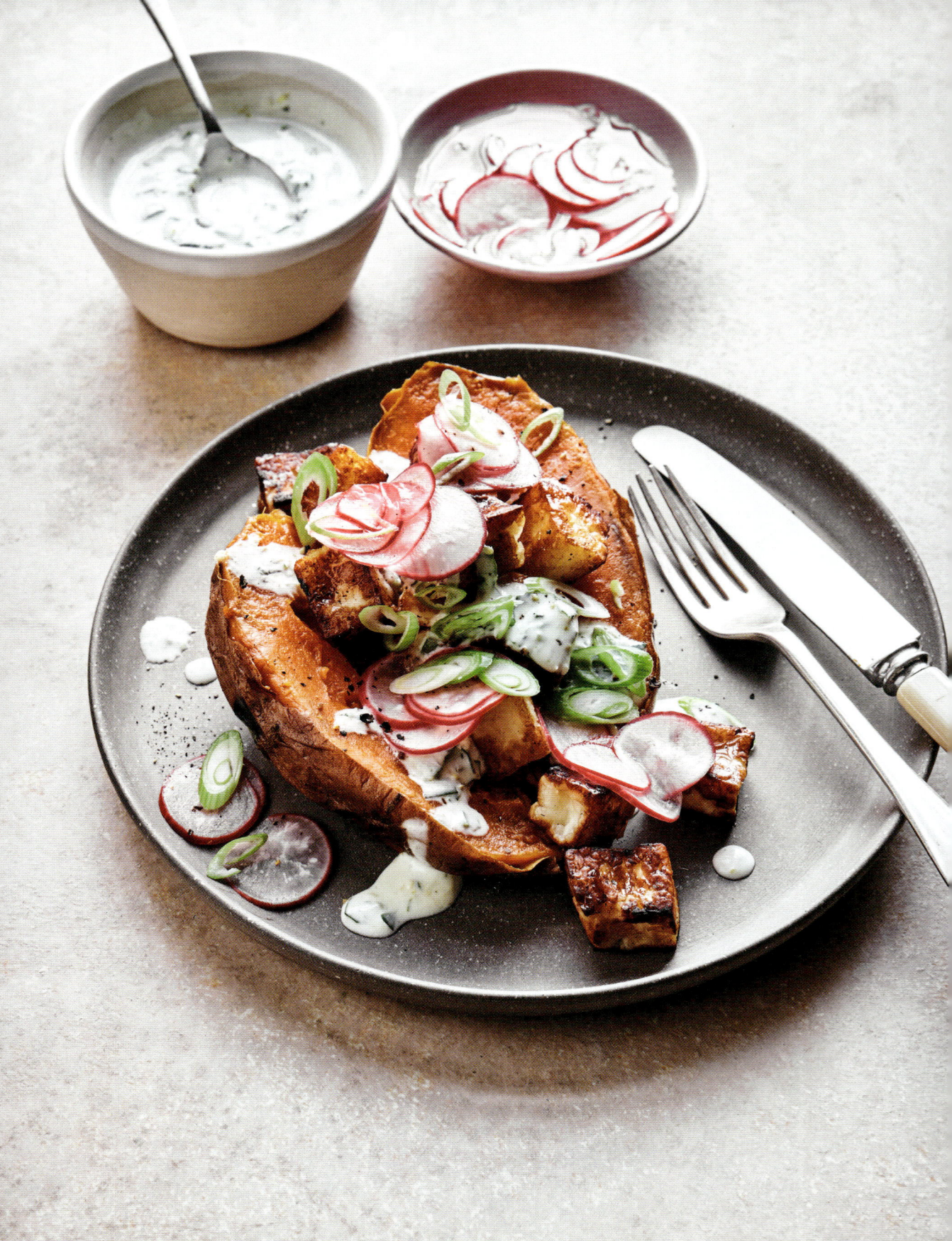

*So simple and easy; microwaving the sweet potato speeds up the baking time while you prep the rest of the ingredients, making this the perfect speedy lunch. Salty, sticky halloumi, pickled radishes and a creamy basil yogurt make this vegetarian dish feel ultra satisfying. Prep and keep the radishes and yogurt in the refrigerator for up to 4 days, and feel free to swap in prawns (shrimp), chicken or tofu in place of halloumi.*

# Halloumi Sweet Potato Jackets with Basil Yogurt

**SERVES 1**
**Under 570kcal,**
**27g protein per serving**

1 fist-sized sweet potato (around 130g/4½oz)

A little olive oil

100ml (scant ½ cup) white vinegar (or rice vinegar)

50ml (3½ tablespoons) water

1 teaspoon sugar

A few handfuls of radishes, thinly sliced into rounds

2 tablespoons Greek yogurt (0% or full fat)

1 teaspoon pesto

Small handful of basil, leaves picked and stems chopped (keep separate)

Zest and juice of 1 lemon

60g (2¼oz) halloumi cheese, cut into cubes

1 small teaspoon honey

1 spring onion (scallion), finely chopped

Salt and pepper

Preheat the oven to 200°C/180°C fan (400°F) Gas Mark 6, or the air fryer to 180°C (350°F). Rub the sweet potato with a little olive oil and season the skin with salt. Stab carefully with a knife, then microwave for about 5 minutes before baking or air frying for another 5–10 minutes, until soft. If just baking, pop it in the oven for 25–30 minutes.

Mix the vinegar, water and sugar together in a bowl. Add the sliced radishes and leave to pickle for at least 15 minutes.

In another bowl, mix the yogurt with the pesto, basil leaves, lemon zest and juice, and season with salt and pepper.

Pan-fry the halloumi with the honey and basil stems over a medium heat until golden brown and sticky, taking care the honey doesn't burn, about 5 minutes.

To serve, cut open the sweet potato and load it with the freshly seared halloumi. Top with a drizzle of the basil yogurt, a scattering of pickled radishes and the spring onion.

*One of my most popular lunch recipes, these chicken crunch bagels have become a staple for so many of you, and I can totally understand why. They're packed full of protein, fibre and energising nutrition, and ready in under 10 minutes.*

# Spicy Chicken Crunch Bagels

**SERVES 2**

**Under 400kcal,**

**30g protein per serving**

½ red (bell) pepper, deseeded and diced

¼ red onion, finely diced

160–200g (5¾–7oz) cooked chicken breast, shredded

2 heaped tablespoons Greek yogurt (0% or full fat)

1 teaspoon wholegrain mustard

Handful of chopped dill

½ jalapeño pepper from a jar, diced

Few dashes of Tabasco

2 wholegrain bagels

50g (1¾oz) feta cheese, crumbled

Salt and pepper

Preheat the oven to 220°C/200°C fan (425°F) Gas Mark 7 on the grill (broiler) setting, or your air fryer to 200°C (400°F).

Place the diced pepper and red onion in a mixing bowl. Add he shredded chicken, yogurt, mustard, dill, jalapeño and salt and pepper to taste. Mix well to combine and taste, adding a few dashes of Tabasco and adjusting the seasoning if needed.

Slice each bagel in half horizontally and evenly spread the chicken mixture on each side. Top with the crumbled feta.

Either cook in the oven for 6–8 minutes or air fry for 6 minutes, until the feta is golden.

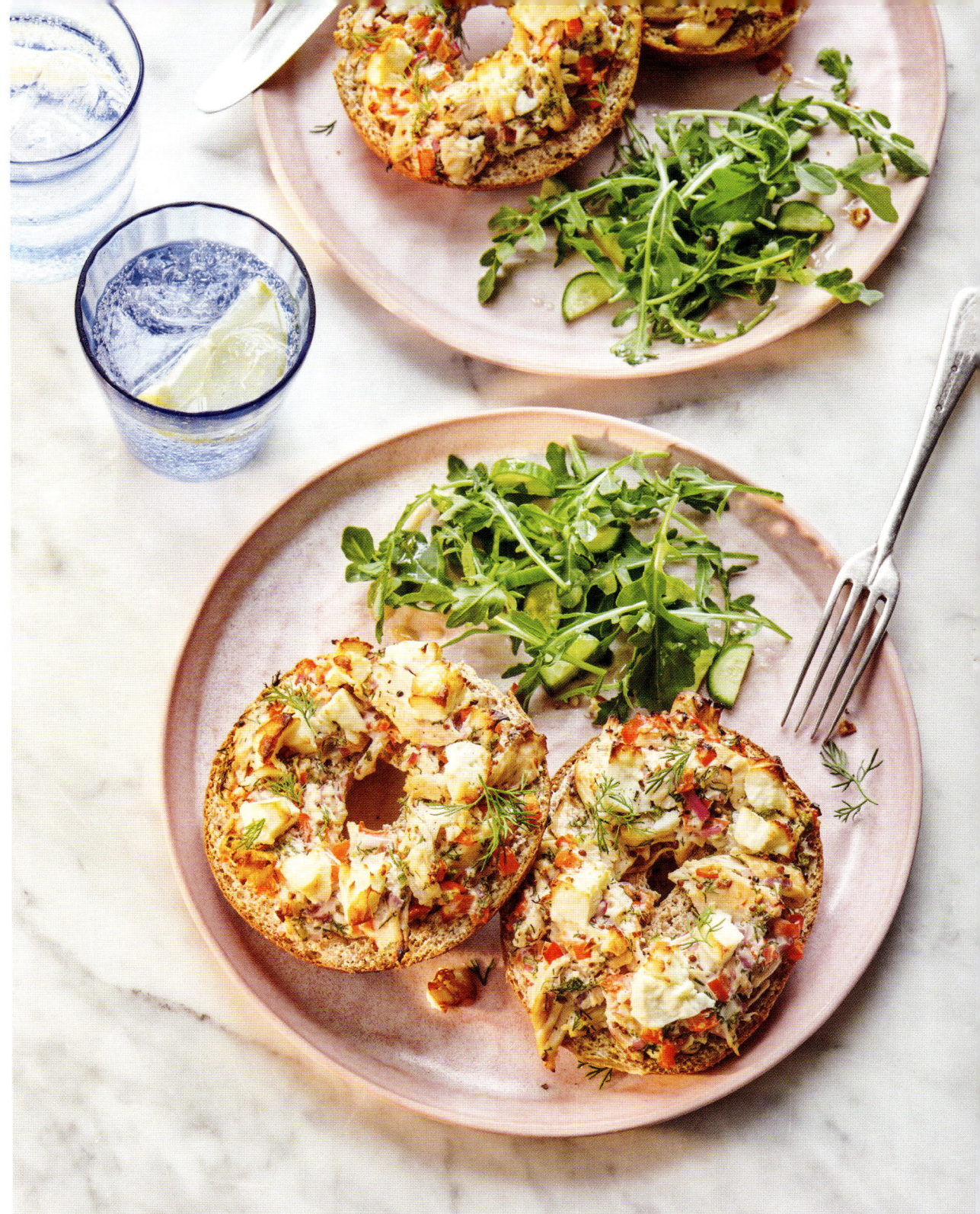

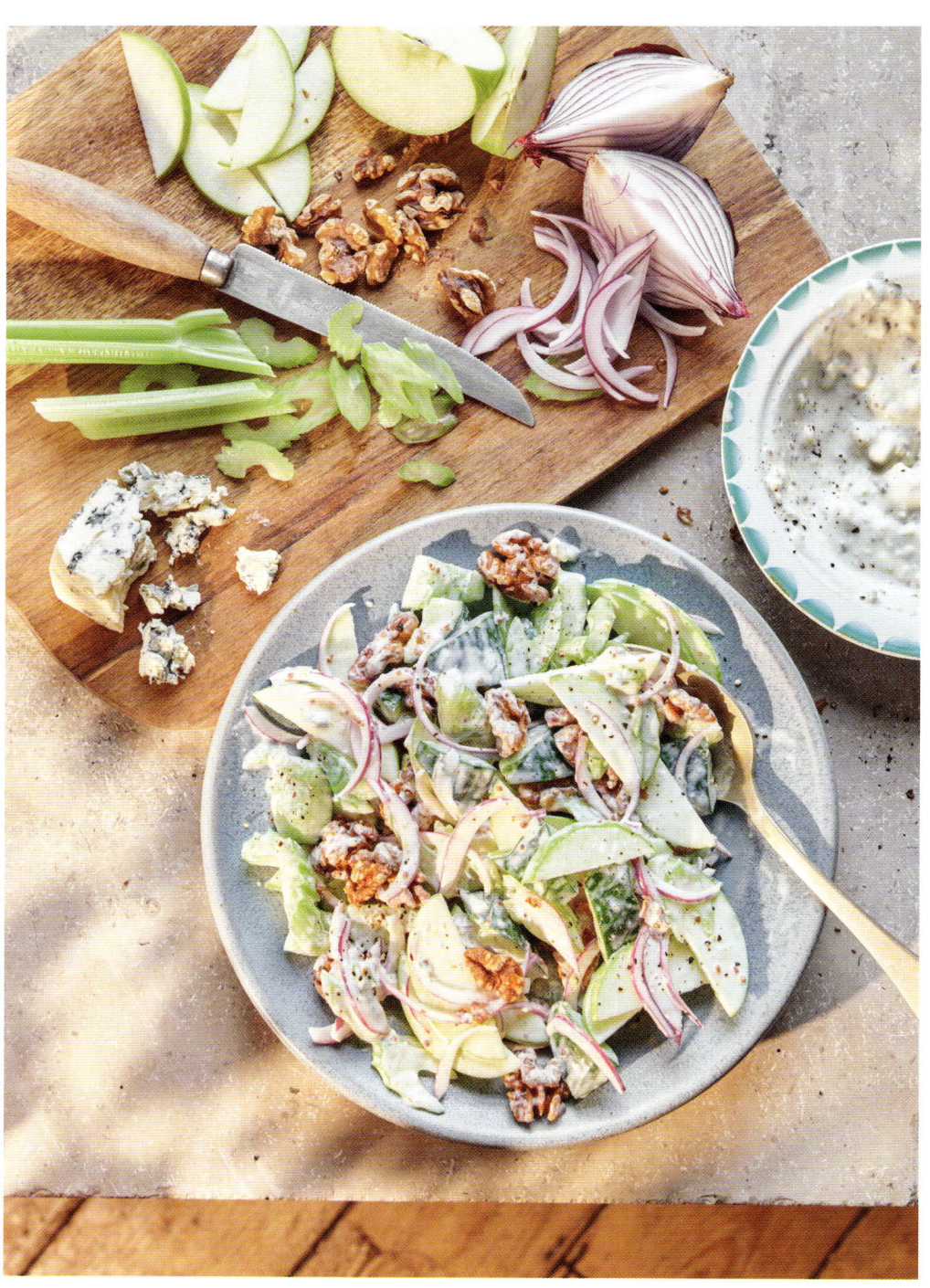

*Anyone who thinks salads are dull and boring needs to try this; it's a perfect combination of creamy, tangy, crunchy, sweet and salty. The salad base contains fresh apple, celery and smashed cucumber, which cling to all the gorgeous dressing. The dressing, made with blue cheese, honey, yogurt, mustard and lemon, brings everything together beautifully. Toss with toasted walnuts, add your preferred protein and serve.*

# Chopped Waldorf Salad

**SERVES 2**
**Under 393kcal,**
**13g protein per serving**

30g (¼ cup) walnut halves

½ cucumber

80g (2¾oz) blue cheese

1 heaped teaspoon wholegrain mustard

1 teaspoon honey

1 heaped tablespoon yogurt

Juice of 1 lemon, plus extra if needed

1 green apple, cored and finely sliced (skin on)

2 celery sticks, finely sliced

½ red onion, finely sliced

200g (7oz) cooked protein, such as shredded roast chicken (not included in macros))

Salt and pepper

Crush the walnuts roughly using your hands and toast them in a dry frying pan over a medium heat for 3–4 minutes until aromatic, tossing regularly and watching they don't burn.

Cut the cucumber in half lengthways. Use a rolling pin to bash each half, then cut into segments.

Crumble the blue cheese into a large bowl. Add the mustard, honey, yogurt and lemon juice, and season with salt and pepper. Roughly mix to form the dressing.

Toss the apple, celery, cucumber, red onion, protein of choice and walnuts into the dressing until well coated. Season to taste with extra lemon juice, salt and pepper if necessary. This will hold really well, making it a great prep-friendly recipe you can take into the office.

*I love how robust and satisfying a good slaw is. I have this on its own, with extra protein in as a lunch, or it's great for making as a big sharing side for dinners and barbecues. It retains its crunch and flavour for days, and the combination of creamy tahini, sweet oranges and crunchy vegetables makes it ideal for warm weather. Enjoy it fresh or as leftovers – it tastes just as good the next day.*

# Sticky Cashew Orange Slaw

**SERVES 4**
**Under 240kcal,**
**6g protein per serving**

½ white cabbage

2 large carrots

4 spring onions (scallions), chopped

1 large orange, peeled and segmented

100g (3½oz) edamame beans or peas (cooked)

Large handful of coriander (cilantro), chopped (or use parsley)

Protein of choice, such as chicken, prawns (shrimp), tofu, aiming for around 80g (2¾oz) per person (optional)

30g (¼ cup) cashew nuts

Salt (optional)

**FOR THE DRESSING**

2 tablespoons toasted sesame oil

2 teaspoons honey

Juice of ½ orange

4 tablespoons light soy sauce

2 tablespoons rice vinegar

1 teaspoon ginger paste

1 teaspoon garlic granules

Pinch of dried chilli flakes

Finely shred the cabbage using a mandoline or knife, and julienne or grate the carrots (I use a julienne peeler). Mix the cabbage, carrots, spring onions, orange, edamame beans or peas and coriander in a large bowl. Incorporate any protein of choice, if using.

For the dressing, whisk together all the ingredients in a small bowl until smooth. Pour it over the salad and toss to coat evenly. Allow it to sit for 5 minutes for the flavours to combine.

Meanwhile, toast the cashew nuts in a dry frying pan over a medium heat for 3–5 minutes until aromatic and golden.

Taste and season the slaw with salt if needed, and feel free to add more of the dressing ingredients to make it sweeter or saltier. Sprinkle with toasted cashew nuts for extra crunch. Serve immediately or store in the refrigerator for up to 3 days.

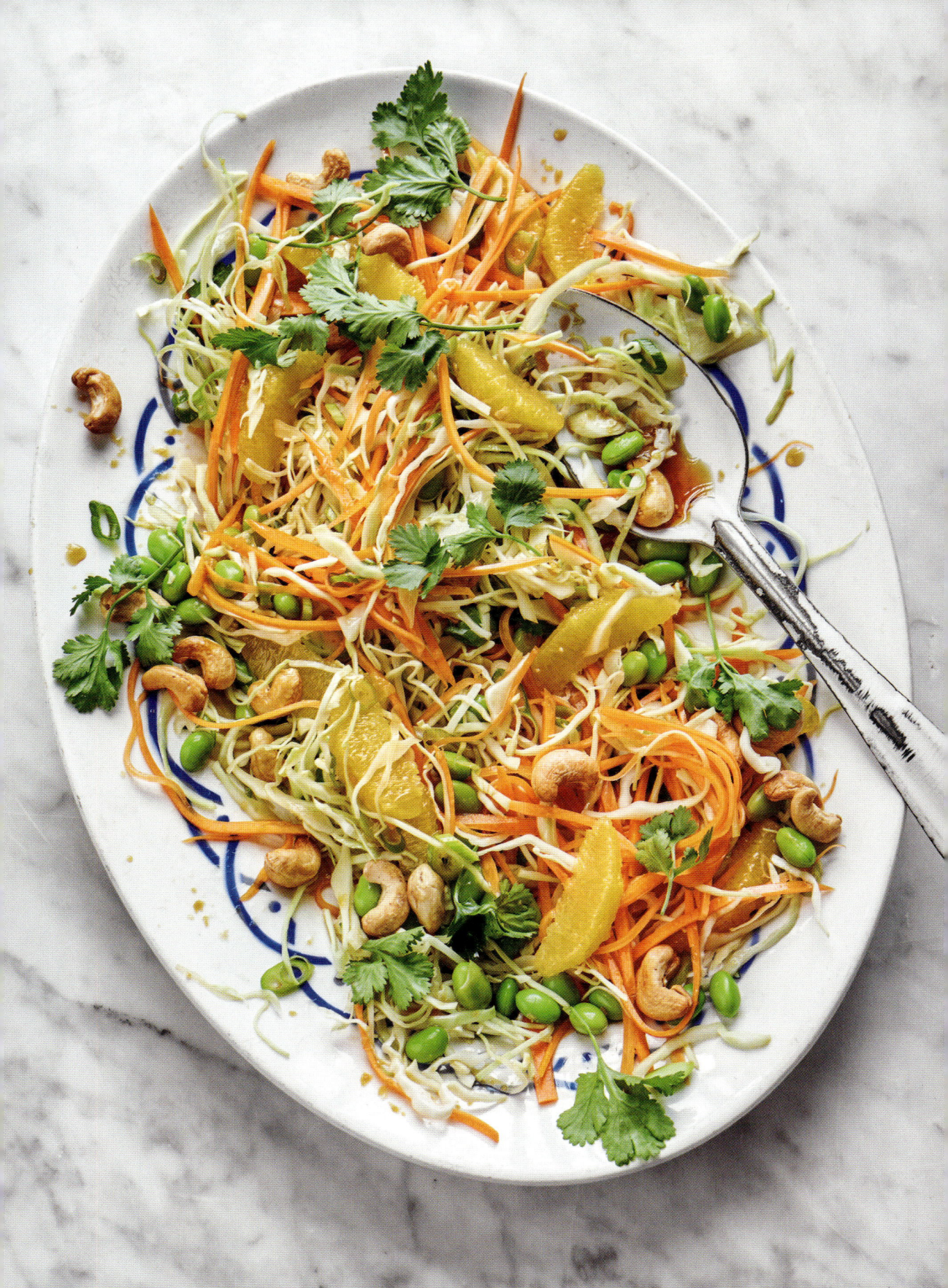

*This recipe is incredibly simple and packed with nutrition, making it the perfect choice for a quick, hearty meal. It's loaded with vibrant greens and has a creamy texture and protein boost from the silken tofu and feta cheese. You'll love how easy it is to prepare, and the flavour is unbeatable. It's perfect for keeping your immune system strong, and it's versatile enough to pair with sourdough toast or shredded chicken for an extra protein hit.*

# Super Greens and Feta Soup

**SERVES 4**
**Under 200kcal,**
**15g protein per serving**

Olive oil, for cooking

1 leek, trimmed, cleaned and sliced

2 celery sticks, chopped

2 garlic cloves, minced

1 head of broccoli, chopped into florets

1 courgette (zucchini), chopped

1 stock cube of choice (I use chicken)

1 teaspoon Dijon mustard

100g (3½oz) baby spinach leaves

300g (10½oz) silken tofu, drained and diced

100g (3½oz) feta cheese, crumbled

2 tablespoons chopped basil

Salt and pepper, to taste

In a large pan, heat a little olive oil over a medium heat. Add the leek, celery and garlic, and sauté for about 5 minutes with a pinch of salt until softened and fragrant. Stir in the broccoli and courgette, and cook for another 3–4 minutes to lightly soften the vegetables.

Dissolve the stock cube into 1.2L (5 cups) of water and pour the stock into the pan. Add the Dijon mustard and stir well. Bring the mixture to a gentle simmer.

Once the soup is simmering, add the spinach and silken tofu. Stir gently until the spinach wilts, which should take about 2–3 minutes.

Remove the pan from the heat and add the feta and basil. Blend the soup using a hand blender or counter-top blender until smooth and creamy.

Season to taste with salt and pepper. Serve the soup hot, optionally pairing it with shredded chicken or toasted sourdough for a more filling meal. Enjoy!

*Sometimes you just crave a big bowl of pasta, and this recipe is perfect for satisfying those cravings. It's balanced, wonderfully filling, and packed with a variety of flavours and nutrients. It's a comforting dish that's quick and easy to whip up for a midweek dinner.*

# Creamy Broccoli and Basil Pasta

**SERVES 2**

**Under 530kcal,**
**50g protein per serving**

150g (5½oz) uncooked pasta of your choice (I like penne or fusilli)

Olive oil, for cooking

1 red onion, finely chopped

1 leek, trimmed, cleaned and finely sliced

2 garlic cloves, minced

1 tablespoon chopped basil stems (plus a handful of torn basil leaves)

1 head of broccoli, chopped into florets

1 chicken stock pot or cube

1 heaped tablespoon light cream cheese

1 tablespoon American mustard

200g (7oz) cooked chicken breast, shredded

50g (1¾oz) Parmesan cheese, grated, plus extra to serve

Salt and pepper, to taste

Cook the pasta in a pan of salted boiling water, according to the packet instructions. Drain, reserving a cup of starchy pasta cooking water, and set aside.

Meanwhile, add a little olive oil to a pan over a medium heat and sauté the red onion, leek and garlic for 4–5 minutes, until softened. Add the chopped basil stems and cook for another minute to enhance the flavour. Add the broccoli florets to the pan and sauté for 2–3 minutes.

Dissolve the chicken stock pot in 150ml (⅔ cup) hot water and pour into the pan. Simmer the vegetables for 5 minutes, until the broccoli is tender but still slightly crisp.

Stir in the light cream cheese and American mustard, mixing until fully incorporated into the sauce. Season generously with black pepper.

Add the shredded chicken and torn basil leaves to the pan, stirring to combine and heating through for about 3 minutes.

Stir in the Parmesan and adjust the seasoning to taste. Toss the pasta into the pan, mixing well to coat in the creamy sauce. Loosen with a little of the pasta cooking water, if necessary.

Divide between two bowls and garnish with extra Parmesan before serving.

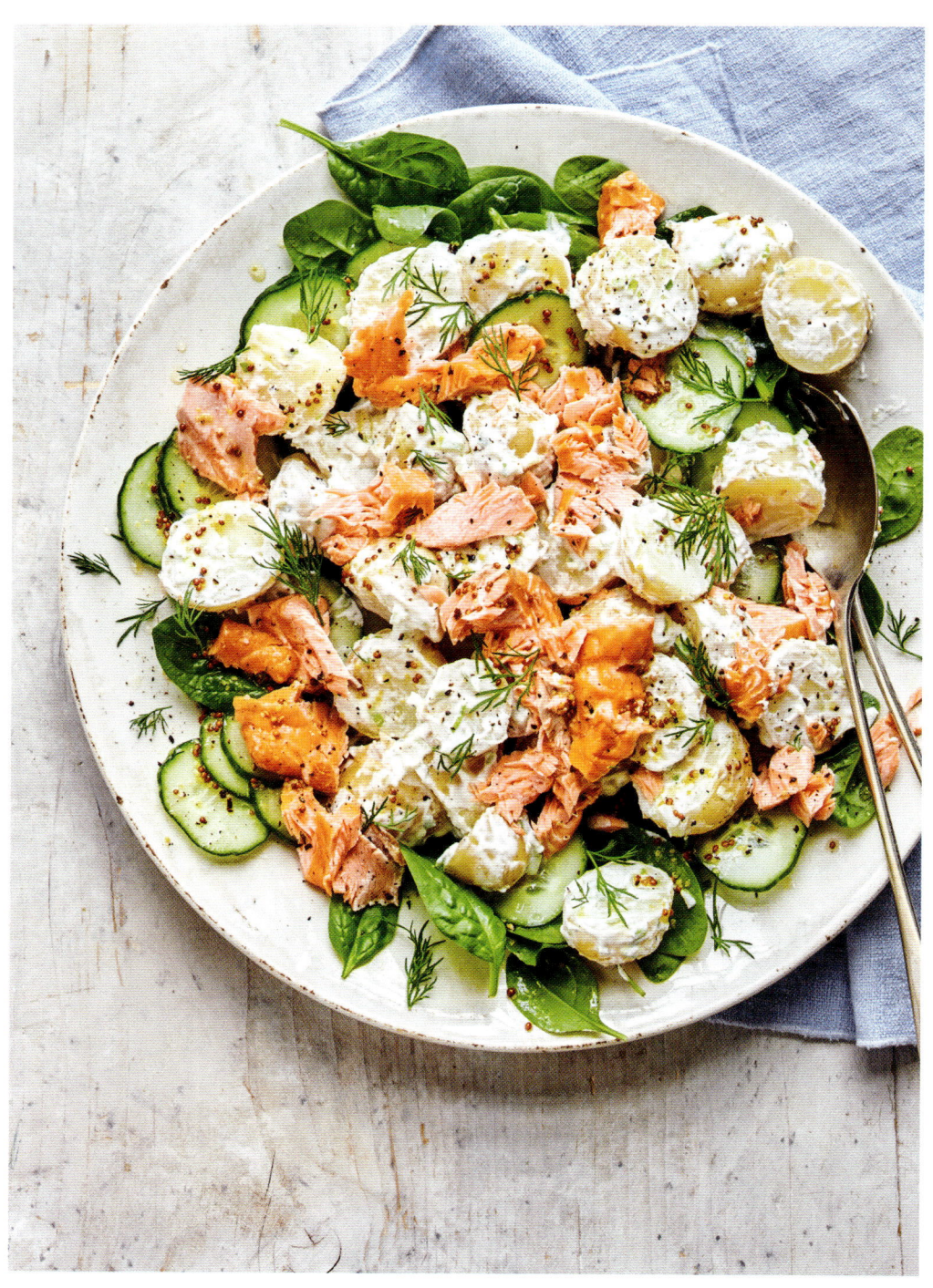

# Hot Smoked Salmon Potato Salad with Vinaigrette

**SERVES 2**
**Under 455kcal,**
**28g protein per serving**

400g (14oz) baby potatoes

3 tablespoons Greek yogurt (0% or full fat)

1 scant teaspoon garlic granules

2 spring onions (scallions), finely chopped, plus extra (optional) to garnish

100g (3½oz) baby spinach leaves

½ cucumber, thinly sliced

2 skinless hot smoked salmon fillets

Salt and pepper

Chopped dill or parsley, to garnish (optional)

**FOR THE VINAIGRETTE**

2 teaspoons olive oil

1 teaspoon Dijon or wholegrain mustard

1 tablespoon honey

Juice of ½ lemon

Cut the baby potatoes into halves or quarters, depending on size. Place into cold salted water and bring up to a gentle simmer for 10–15 minutes, until tender. Drain and set aside.

In a large bowl, combine the yogurt, garlic granules and spring onions. Season with salt and pepper, add the cooked potatoes and toss to coat evenly.

In a small bowl, whisk together the vinaigrette ingredients until well combined. Season with salt and pepper to taste.

Layer the spinach and sliced cucumber on a large serving plate or in a bowl, and add the potato mixture on top. Place the hot smoked salmon on top of the salad and drizzle over the vinaigrette.

Garnish with dill or parsley, if desired. Serve immediately or store in the refrigerator for up to 3 days.

*These tarts will bring a smile to anyone's face; they look beautiful but are easy to make. Using a sheet of ready-rolled puff pastry, the ricotta filling is mixed with feta, basil, spring onion, lemon zest and garlic, creating a creamy and flavourful base. The tarts are topped with seasoned sliced tomatoes and baked until golden.*

# Tomato Tarts with Herby Feta and Ricotta

**SERVES 4**
**Under 412kcal,**
**12g protein per serving**

200g (7oz) ready-
    rolled puff pastry
250g (1 cup) ricotta cheese
100g (3½oz) feta
    cheese, crumbled
Large handful of basil
    leaves, chopped
2 spring onions (scallions),
    finely chopped
Zest of 1 lemon
1 teaspoon garlic granules
4–6 large vine tomatoes,
    sliced (I also like to
    use heritage tomatoes
    when in season)
Olive oil, for glazing
Salt and pepper

**FOR THE SIDE SALAD**
Mixed salad leaves
1 tablespoon olive oil
1 tablespoon balsamic vinegar

Preheat the oven to 220°C/200°C fan (425°F) Gas Mark 7.

Cut the pastry sheet into 4 individual rectangles, about 10 x 15cm (4 x 6 inches) each. Place on a baking tray lined with nonstick baking paper, then score a 1cm (½ inch) border around each rectangle, being careful not to cut all the way through.

In a bowl, combine the ricotta, feta, basil, spring onions, lemon zest and garlic granules. Season with salt and pepper to taste and mix until well combined.

Spread the ricotta mixture evenly within the scored borders of each pastry rectangle. Layer the sliced tomatoes over the ricotta filling, slightly overlapping them. Season the tomatoes with salt and pepper and lightly brush the edges of the puff pastry with olive oil.

Bake in the oven for 15–20 minutes or until the pastry is puffed and golden brown.

While the tarts are baking, prepare the side salad by tossing the mixed salad leaves with the oil, vinegar and some salt and pepper.

Serve the tomato tarts warm, accompanied by the dressed side salad.

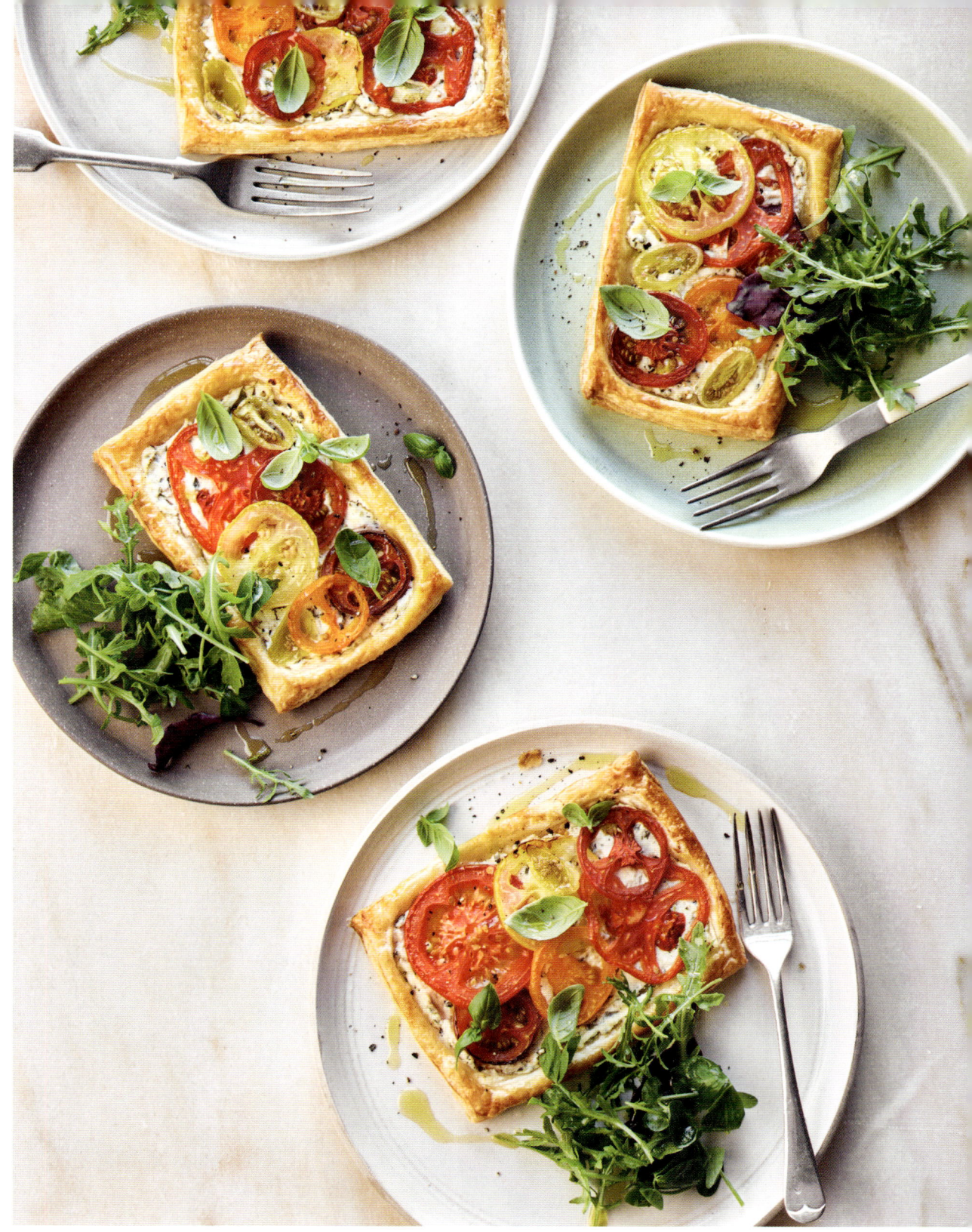

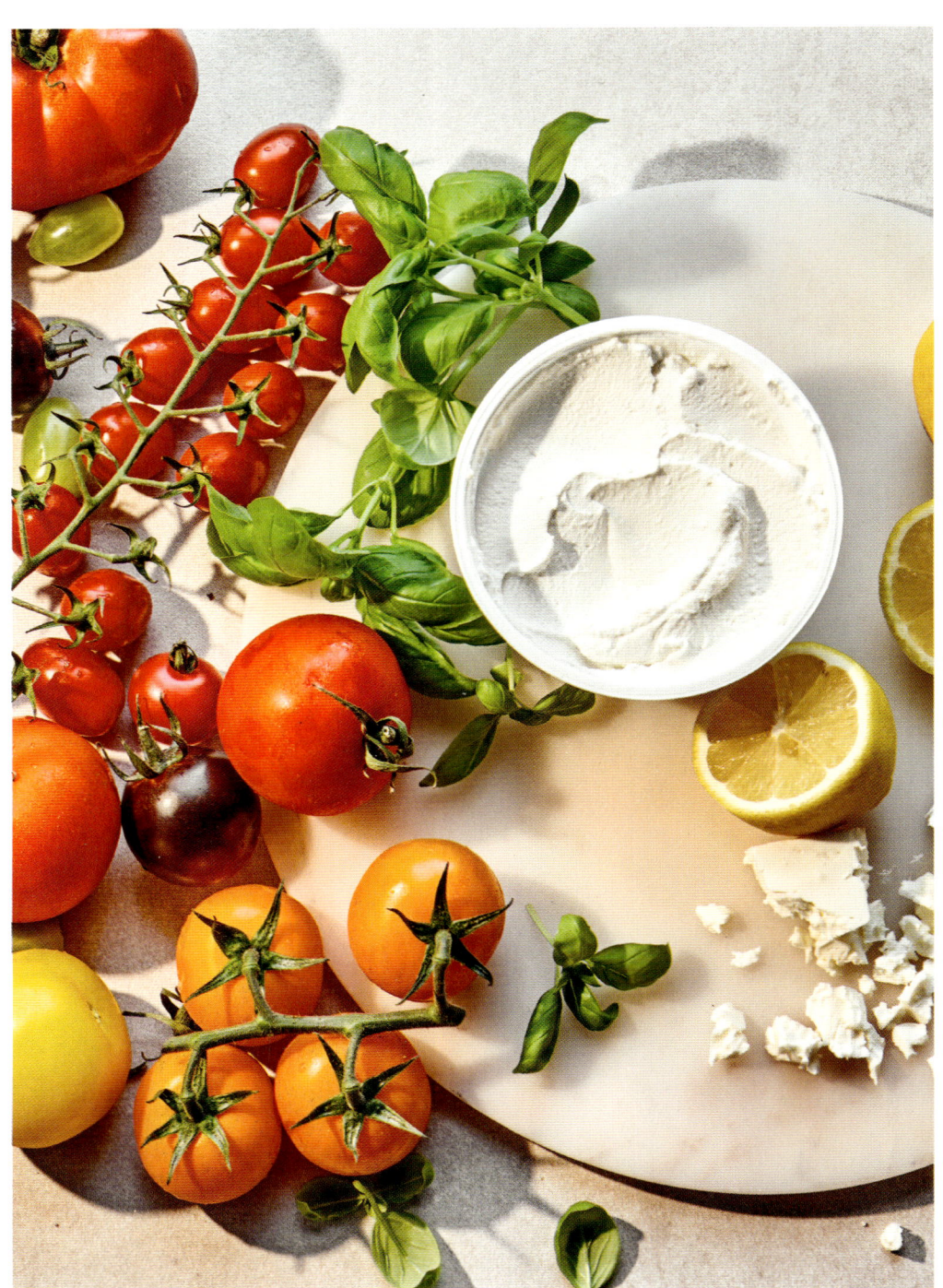

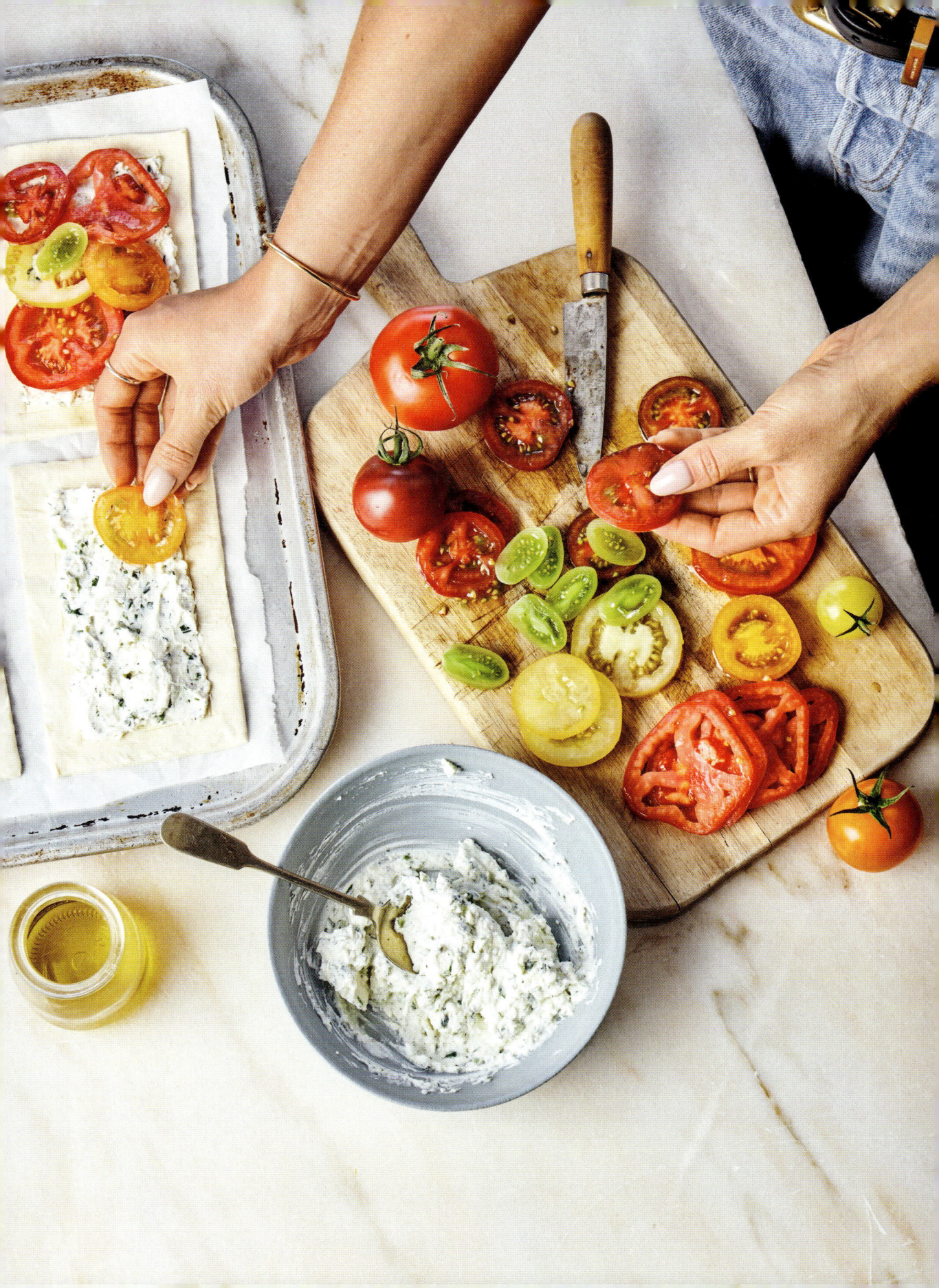

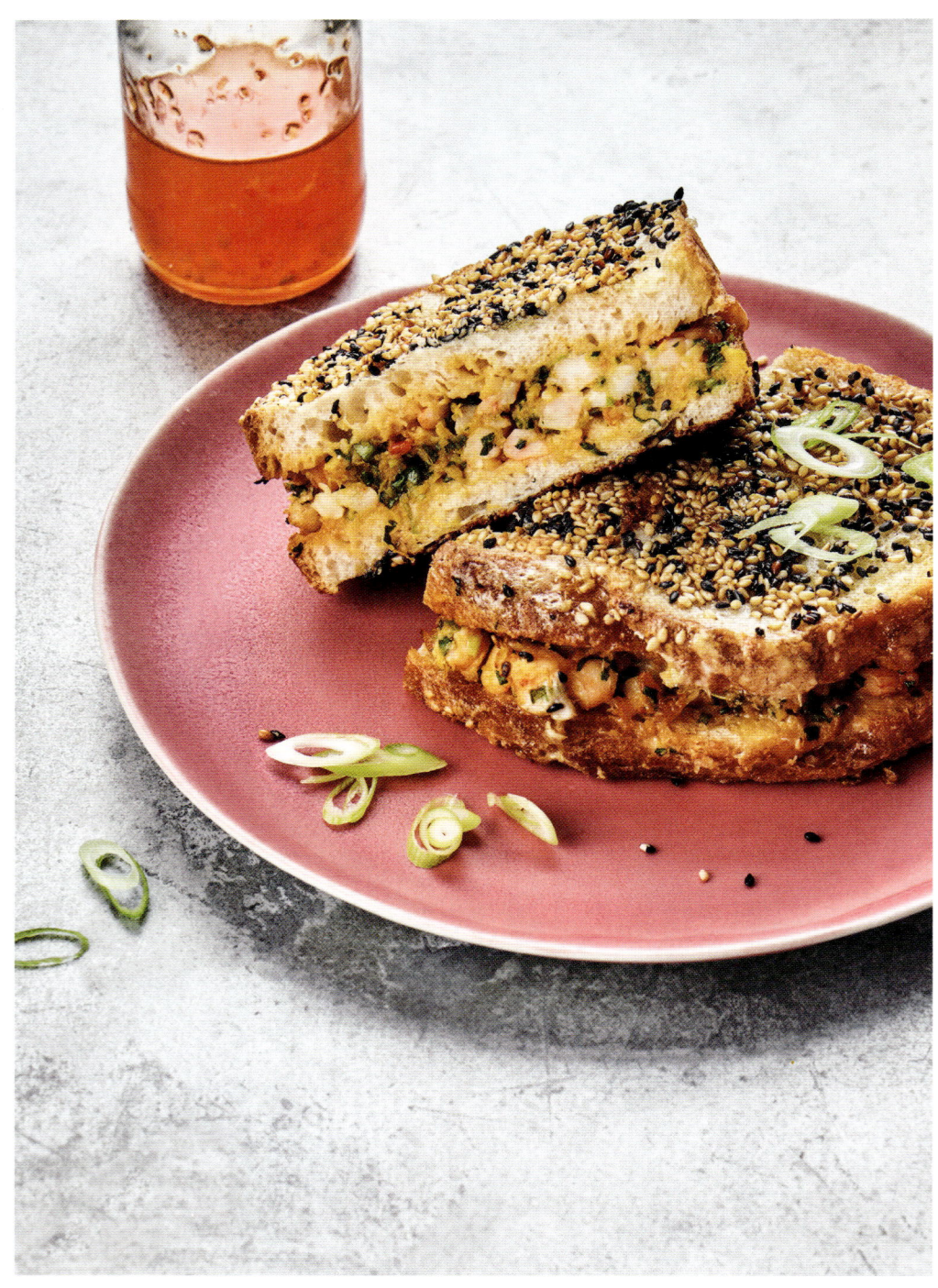

*Taking the flavours of the takeaway classic, this is a quick and tasty upgrade to your typical lunch. It's ready in under 10 minutes and combines high-protein prawns with fresh herbs, crunchy vegetables and a tangy sweet chilli sauce.*

# Prawn Toast Toastie

**SERVES 1**

**Under 300kcal,**
**40g protein per serving**

1 tablespoon chopped parsley or coriander (cilantro), finely chopped

1 spring onion (scallion), finely chopped

100g (3½oz) peeled raw king prawns (shrimp)

2 tablespoons finely grated carrot

½ teaspoon ginger paste

½ teaspoon garlic granules

1 heaped teaspoon sweet chilli sauce, plus extra (optional) to serve

1 tablespoon light soy sauce

Pinch of dried chilli flakes

1 teaspoon toasted sesame oil

1 medium free-range egg, separated

2 slices bread of choice

1 heaped tablespoon sesame seeds, to coat

Neutral oil, for frying

Add the parsley or coriander and spring onion to a bowl.

Mince the prawns by chopping roughly, then running your knife through; some chunky bits are great! Add to a bowl with the grated carrot, ginger paste, garlic granules, sweet chilli sauce, soy sauce, chilli flakes, sesame oil and egg yolk, and mix together.

Spread the filling over one slice of bread, and top with the other; press to seal. Dip the sandwich into the egg white and sprinkle over sesame seeds to coat both sides.

Heat a little oil in a frying pan and sear the sandwich on one side for 3 minutes to colour. Flip, turn the heat down to low, cover the pan with a lid and cook for another 3 minutes; flip again and cook for a final 3 minutes until the filling is cooked through, but watch the sesame seeds don't burn.

Serve with a little extra sweet chilli sauce if you like!

*Quiche is a classic lunchtime staple, and I wanted to give it my signature twist and transform your standard recipe into one full of protein, healthy fats and balanced nutrition. Blending the cottage cheese to form a creamy custard base is the secret here, as well as using light filo layered with olive oil. I like to bake this in a deep cake tin, but you can bake it into individual muffin cases; adjust the cooking time accordingly.*

# Salmon and Spinach Filo Cottage Cheese Quiche

**SERVES 6**
**Under 255kcal,**
**20g protein per serving**

Spray oil, for greasing
300g (1¼ cups) cottage cheese
100ml (scant ½ cup) milk
5 medium free-range eggs
100g (3½oz) baby spinach leaves, wilted and chopped
10g (¼oz) chopped chives
100g (3½oz) smoked salmon, chopped
Zest of 1 lemon
4 sheets of filo (phyllo) pastry, each cut in half
50g (1¾oz) feta cheese, crumbled
Salt and pepper

Preheat the oven to 180°C/160°C fan (350°F) Gas Mark 4. Lightly spray a 20cm (8 inch) deep springform cake tin (pan) with oil.

In a blender or food processor, blend the cottage cheese with the milk until smooth. Transfer to a large mixing bowl. Add the eggs to the bowl and whisk until well combined. Stir in the wilted spinach, chives, smoked salmon, lemon zest and salt and pepper to taste. Mix until all the ingredients are evenly distributed.

Layer the halved filo sheets into the oiled cake tin, spraying each sheet lightly with oil as you go. Ensure the sheets are layered evenly to form a sturdy crust, overlapping to cover any gaps.

Pour the cottage cheese and egg mixture into the prepared filo crust. Tuck the edges of the filo back in on themselves to create a neat edge – you can be rough with this; don't worry about it being perfect. Sprinkle the crumbled feta evenly over the top of the filling.

Bake in the oven for 60 minutes, or until the filling is just set. It will continue to set as it cools, so allow the quiche to cool slightly before serving. This also makes it easier to slice.

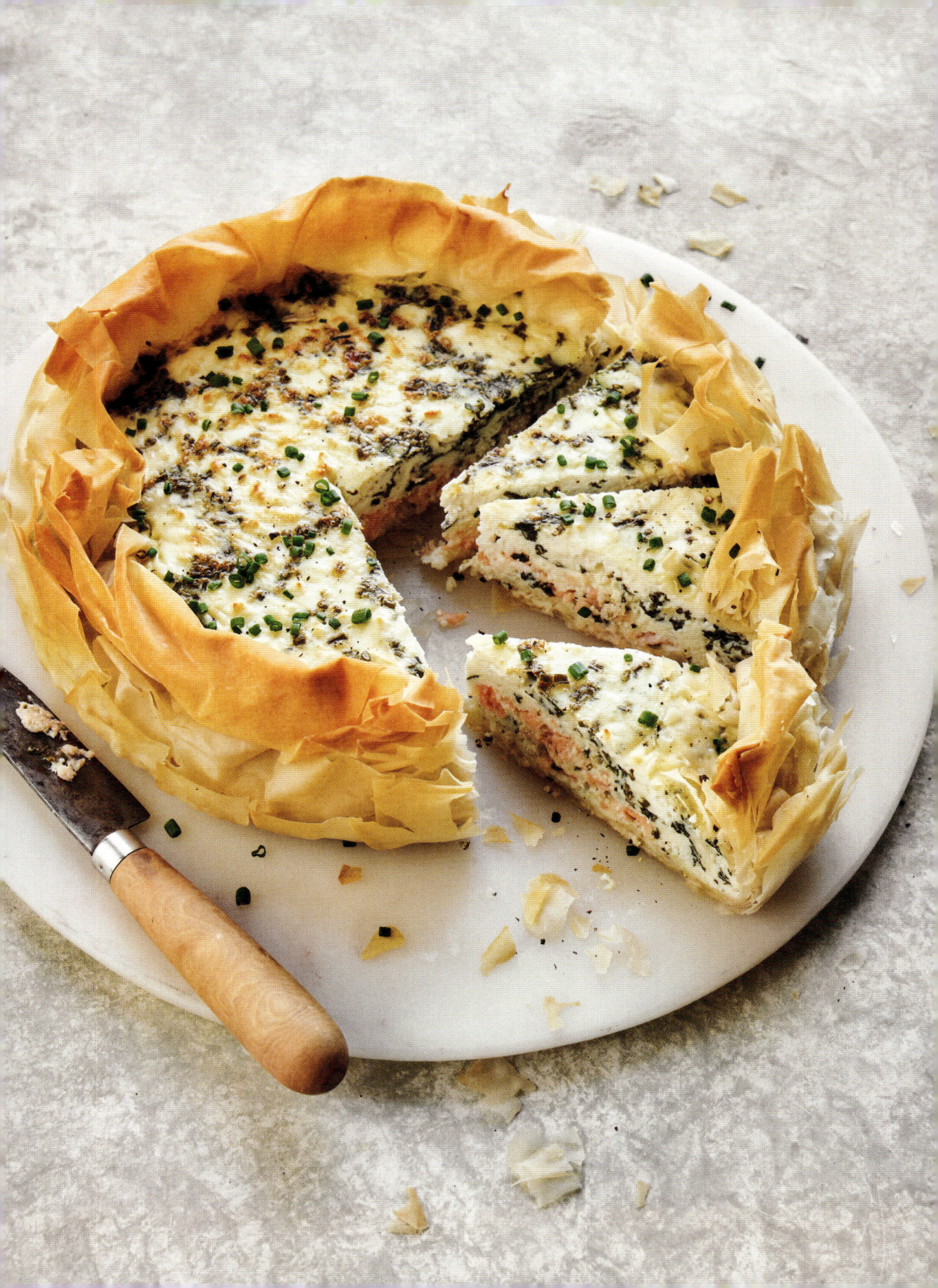

*Once you make a potato salad like this, it's hard to go back. The yogurt and mustard dressing ties everything together beautifully, with the perfect balance of creamy, crunchy, fresh and bright. This dish is quick and easy to prepare, making it a perfect recipe for a wholesome meal, both satisfying and delicious.*

# Crispy Smashed Potato Mackerel Salad

**SERVES 2**
**Under 420kcal,**
**23g protein per serving**

250g (9oz) baby potatoes

Olive oil, for drizzling

20g (¾oz) Parmesan cheese, grated

½ cucumber, deseeded and diced

½ red onion, finely sliced

Small handful of pitted black olives, halved

2 smoked mackerel fillets, skin removed, flaked

1 tablespoon chopped dill or parsley

2 heaped tablespoons Greek yogurt (0% or full fat)

1 teaspoon wholegrain mustard

Zest of 1 lemon and a little juice

Salt and pepper

Preheat the oven to 220°C/200°C fan (425°F) Gas Mark 7.

Bring a large pan of salted water to the boil and add the baby potatoes. Simmer until tender all the way through, then drain and spread across a baking sheet.

Using a mug or flat-bottomed small bowl, press down firmly on each potato to crush them but so they are still holding together. Drizzle over some olive oil, season with salt and pepper and sprinkle over the Parmesan. Bake in the oven for 25–30 minutes, until golden and crisp. Remove and leave to cool slightly.

In a large bowl, mix the cucumber, red onion, olives, flaked mackerel and herbs. Add the crushed potatoes, yogurt, mustard, lemon zest, a little squeeze of juice, some pepper and a pinch of salt. Gently toss everything together to coat evenly, then serve.

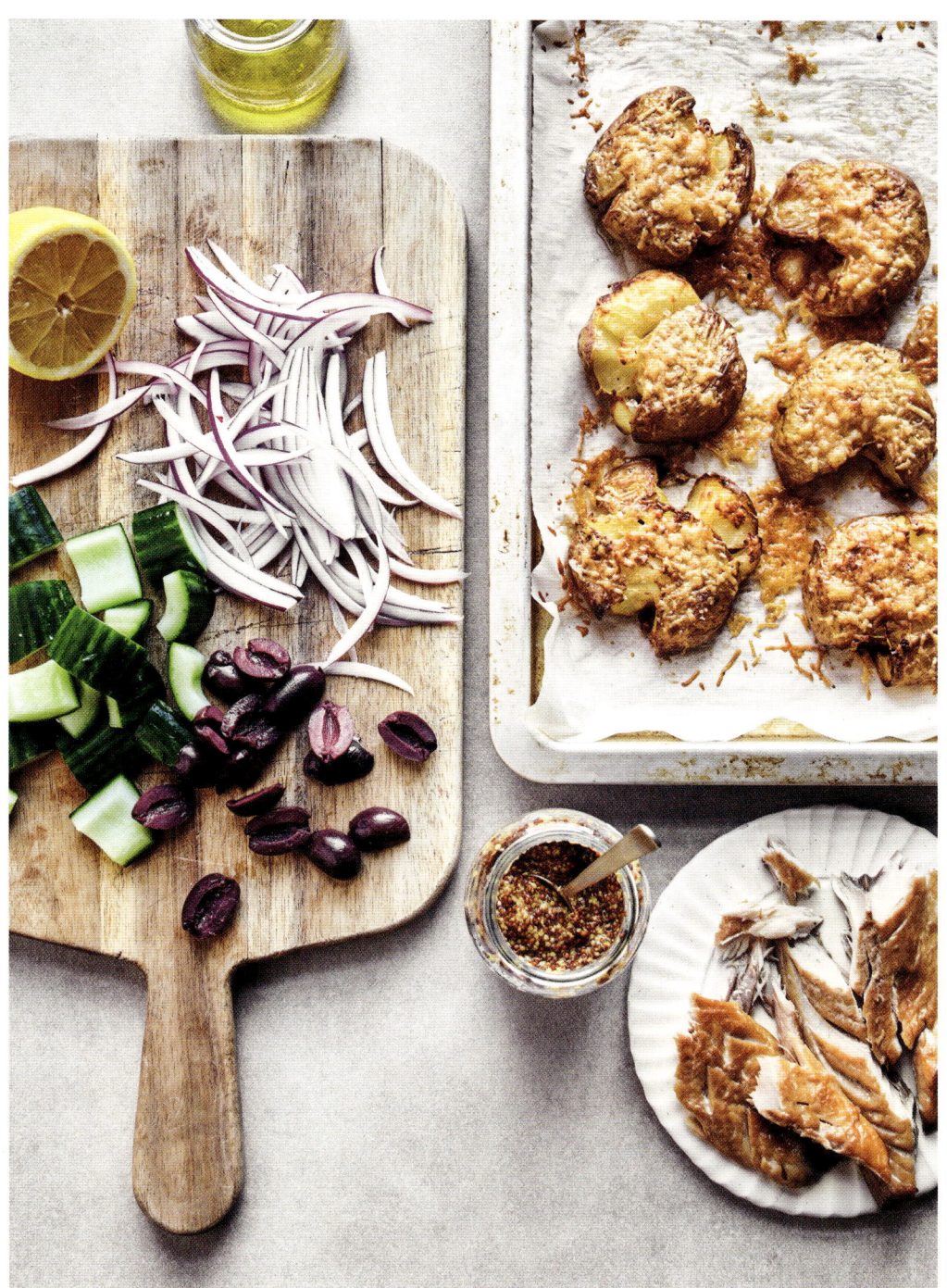

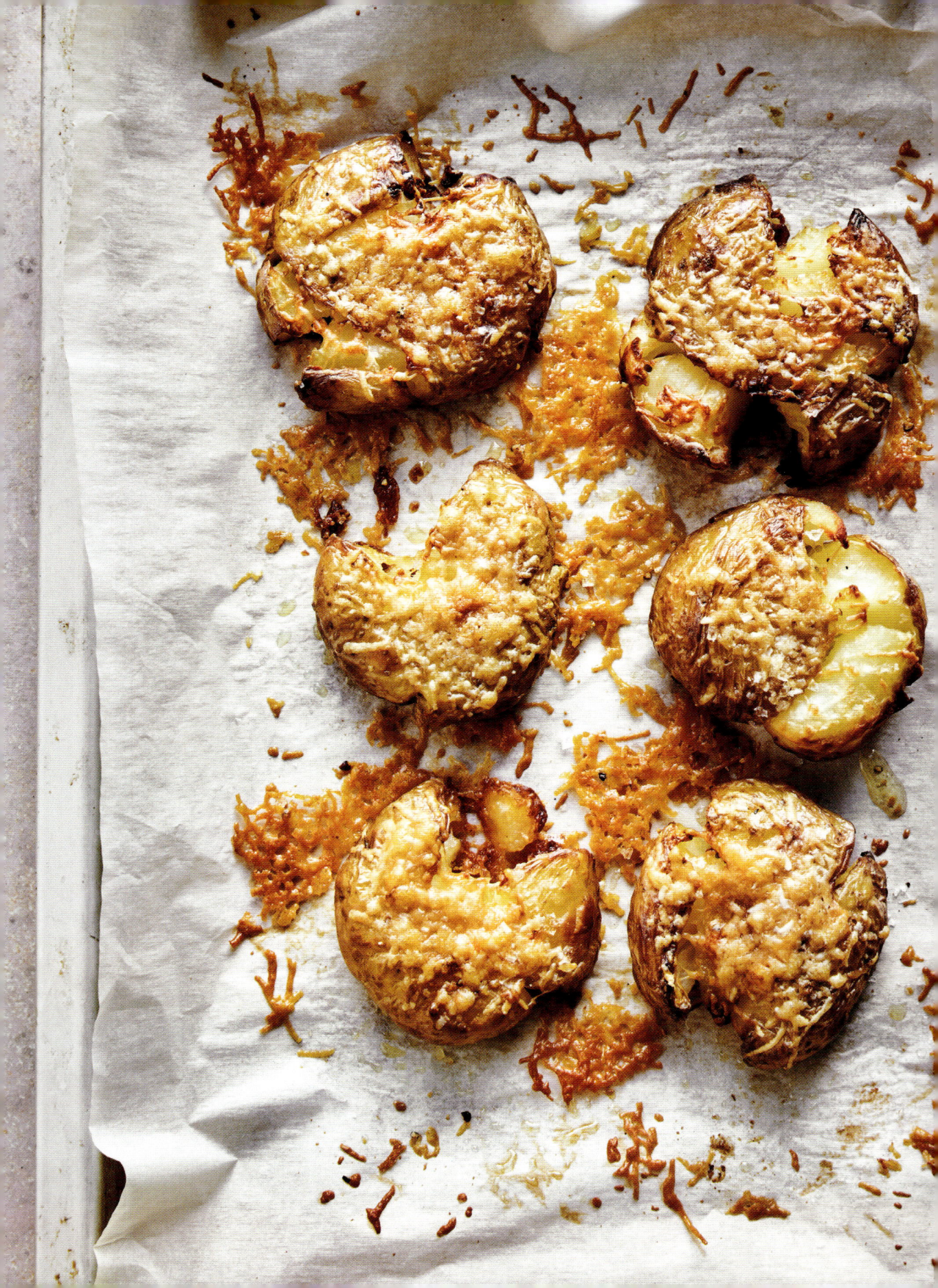

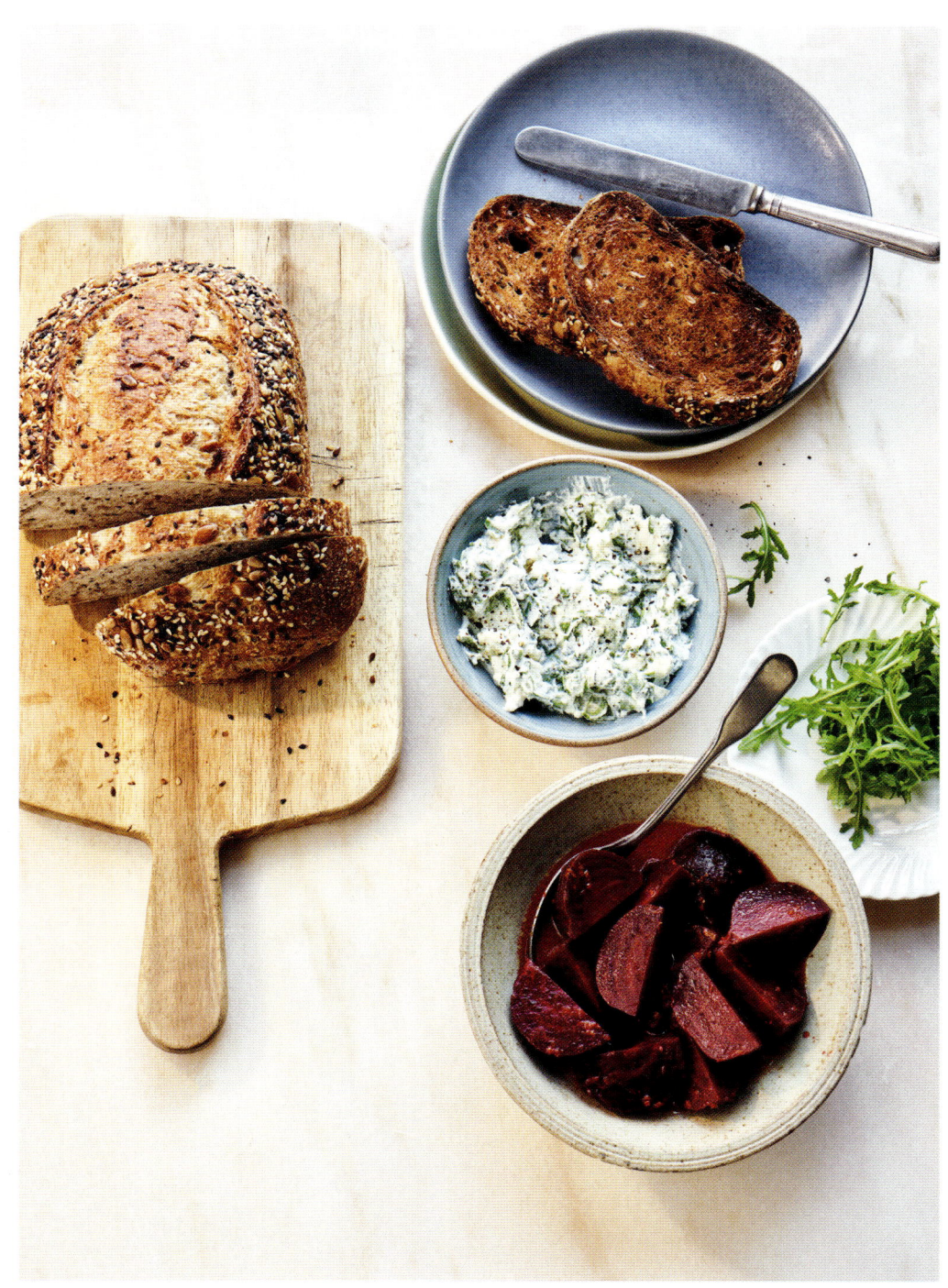

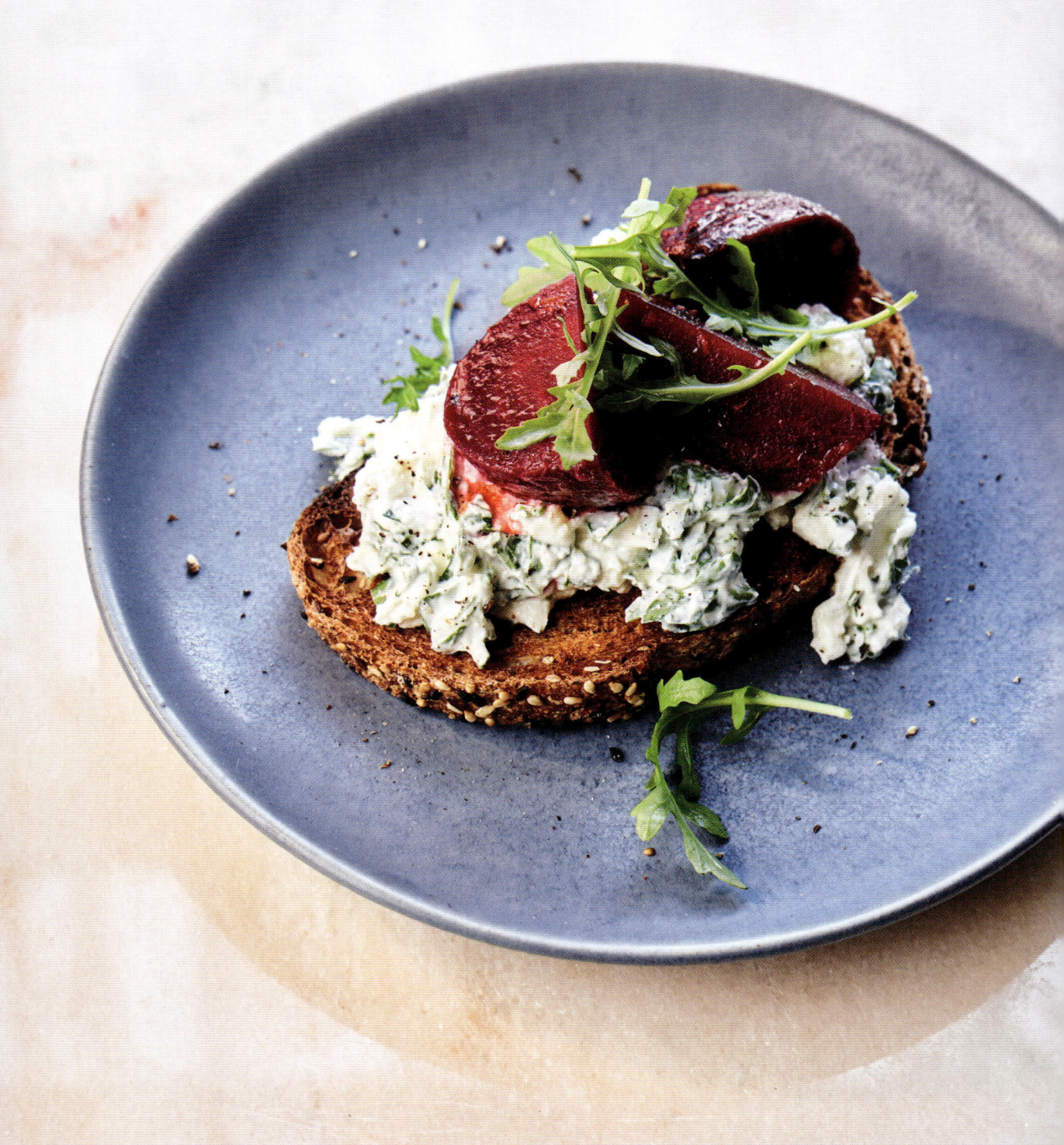

*I always say colour, not calories, and one colour we don't always get enough of is purple. Combining creamy goat's cheese, fresh spinach and marinated beetroot on slices of sourdough, these tartines are perfect for packing in the nutrition, but all on toast. Easy to prepare, the marinated beetroot leftovers are great for adding to salads or other dishes and can be stored in the refrigerator for several days.*

# Spinach, Goat's Cheese and Beetroot Tartine

**SERVES 2**
**Under 384kcal,**
**17g protein per serving**

80g (2¾oz) goat's
  cheese, crumbled
2 heaped tablespoons Greek
  yogurt (0% or full fat)
Handful of baby spinach
  leaves, chopped
½ teaspoon garlic granules
Small pinch of thyme leaves
2 slices of sourdough bread,
  or any bread of choice
Salt and pepper
Handful of rocket
  (arugula), to garnish

**FOR THE BEETROOT**
Zest and juice of 1 orange
1 tablespoon olive oil
1 tablespoon white
  wine vinegar
1 scant teaspoon
  Dijon mustard
1 x 250g (9oz) pack of
  precooked beetroot
  (beets), quartered

In a large bowl, whisk together the orange zest and juice, olive oil, vinegar, mustard and some salt and pepper. Add the beetroot quarters to the marinade and toss to coat. Leave to marinate while you prep the rest of the meal.

In another bowl, combine the goat's cheese, yogurt, spinach, garlic granules and thyme. Season with salt and pepper to taste and mix until well combined.

Toast the bread and spread the goat's cheese mixture evenly over each slice. Top with marinated beetroot quarters and garnish with rocket for a pop of colour and extra flavour.

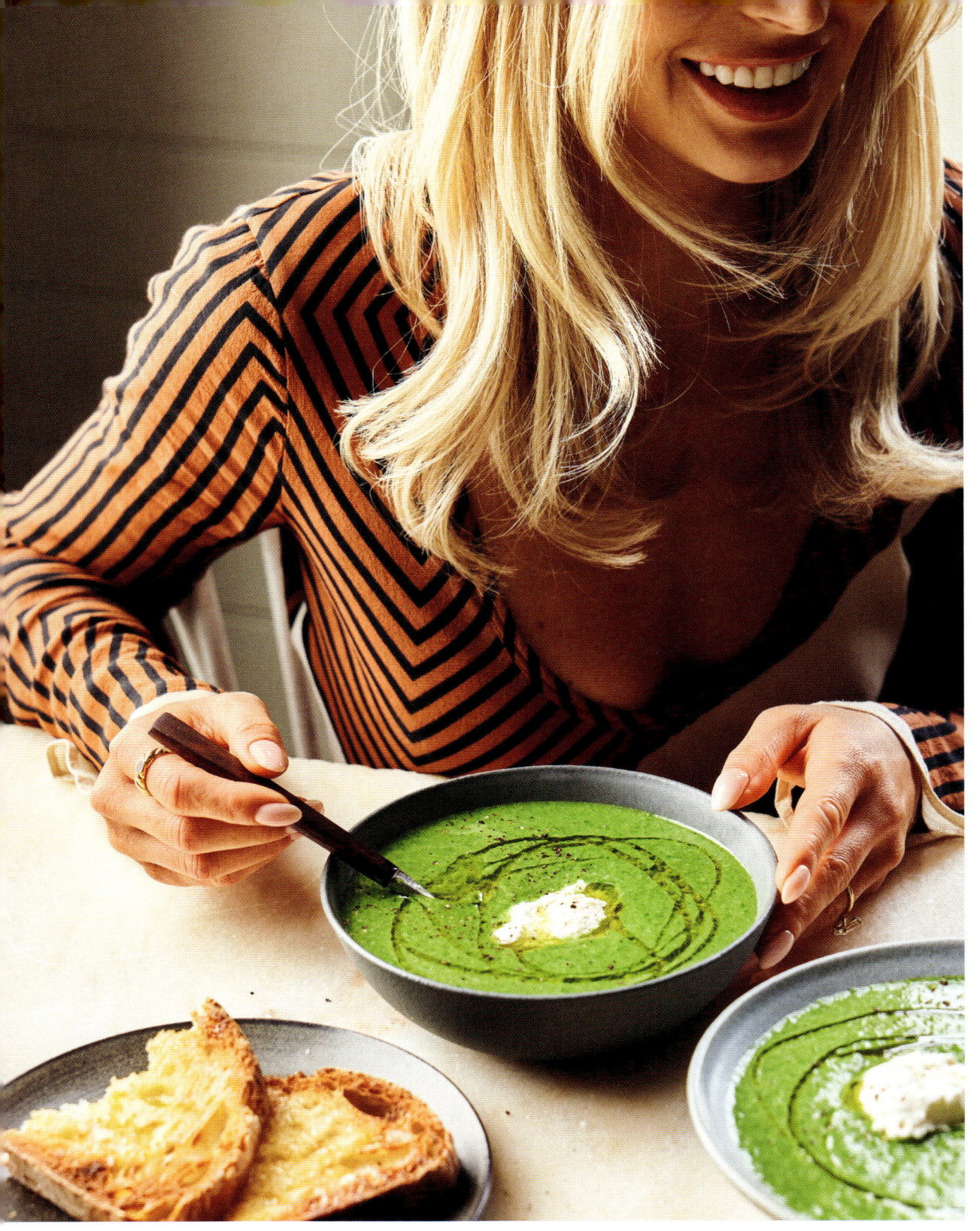

*I love how I can always pack so much goodness into a soup, and this recipe is full of fibre and lots of plant protein to make a filling, nutrient-packed meal. Served with a full dollop of ricotta, it's creamy and unctuous, and belongs with a big slice of bread for dunking.*

# Protein Power Pea and Miso Soup with Whipped Ricotta

**SERVES 4**
**Under 320kcal,**
**18g protein per serving**

1 tablespoon olive oil

1 leek, trimmed, cleaned and sliced

2 garlic cloves, minced

2 celery sticks, chopped

200g (1⅓ cups) frozen peas

200g (7oz) baby spinach leaves

1 x 400g (14oz) can of cannellini beans, drained and rinsed

1 litre (generous 4 cups) chicken or vegetable stock

Handful of basil leaves

1 scant tablespoon white miso

Salt and pepper

**FOR THE WHIPPED LEMON PARMESAN RICOTTA**

250g (1 cup) ricotta cheese

Zest of 1 lemon

1 tablespoon lemon juice

60g (2¼oz) Parmesan cheese, grated

Heat the olive oil in a large pan over a medium heat. Add the leek, garlic and celery and sauté for about 5 minutes, until softened.

Add the frozen peas, spinach and cannellini beans, pour in the stock and bring to the boil. Reduce the heat and let it simmer for 10–15 minutes, or until all the vegetables are tender.

While the soup is simmering, prepare the whipped lemon Parmesan ricotta. In a small bowl, combine the ingredients with salt and pepper to taste. Whip together until smooth and creamy.

Add the basil leaves and miso to the soup pan and use a stick blender to blend until smooth. Season with salt and pepper to taste.

Serve the soup hot, topped with a generous dollop of the whipped ricotta.

*Note: This soup can be stored in the refrigerator for up to 3 days. Reheat gently before serving. The whipped lemon Parmesan ricotta can also be made ahead of time and stored in the refrigerator for up to 3 days.*

*This is one of my go-to recipes when I'm not feeling my best. It's a comforting and nutritious meal that comes together in under 10 minutes, making it perfect for a quick and satisfying lunch.*

# Chicken Sweetcorn Egg Drop Soup

**SERVES 2**
**Under 318kcal,**
**33g protein per serving**

Oil, for cooking

1 large garlic clove, minced

½ teaspoon chopped fresh ginger

2 spring onions (scallions), chopped, plus extra to serve

1.2 litres (5 cups) chicken stock (made from 1 chicken stock cube)

180g (1¼ cups) frozen sweetcorn

Pinch of white pepper

200g (7oz) cooked shredded chicken breast

2 tablespoons light soy sauce, or more to taste

1 heaped tablespoon cornflour (cornstarch) mixed with 3 tablespoons water to form a paste

1 large free-range egg, beaten

Toasted sesame oil or crispy chilli oil, to serve (optional)

Heat a little oil in a pan over a low to medium heat, add the garlic, ginger and spring onions and sweat for a few minutes. Tip in the stock and bring to a simmer. Add the frozen sweetcorn, white pepper, shredded chicken and soy sauce, and bring back to a simmer. Pour in the cornflour paste, stir, and allow to simmer gently for 4–5 minutes until slightly thickened. Feel free to add more cornflour if needed. Taste and season with more soy sauce if you wish.

Take off the heat and slowly pour the beaten egg into the middle of the soup. Allow it to sit for 15 seconds, then slowly stir the soup to form egg ribbons.

Serve with extra spring onion, and some toasted sesame or chilli oil if you like.

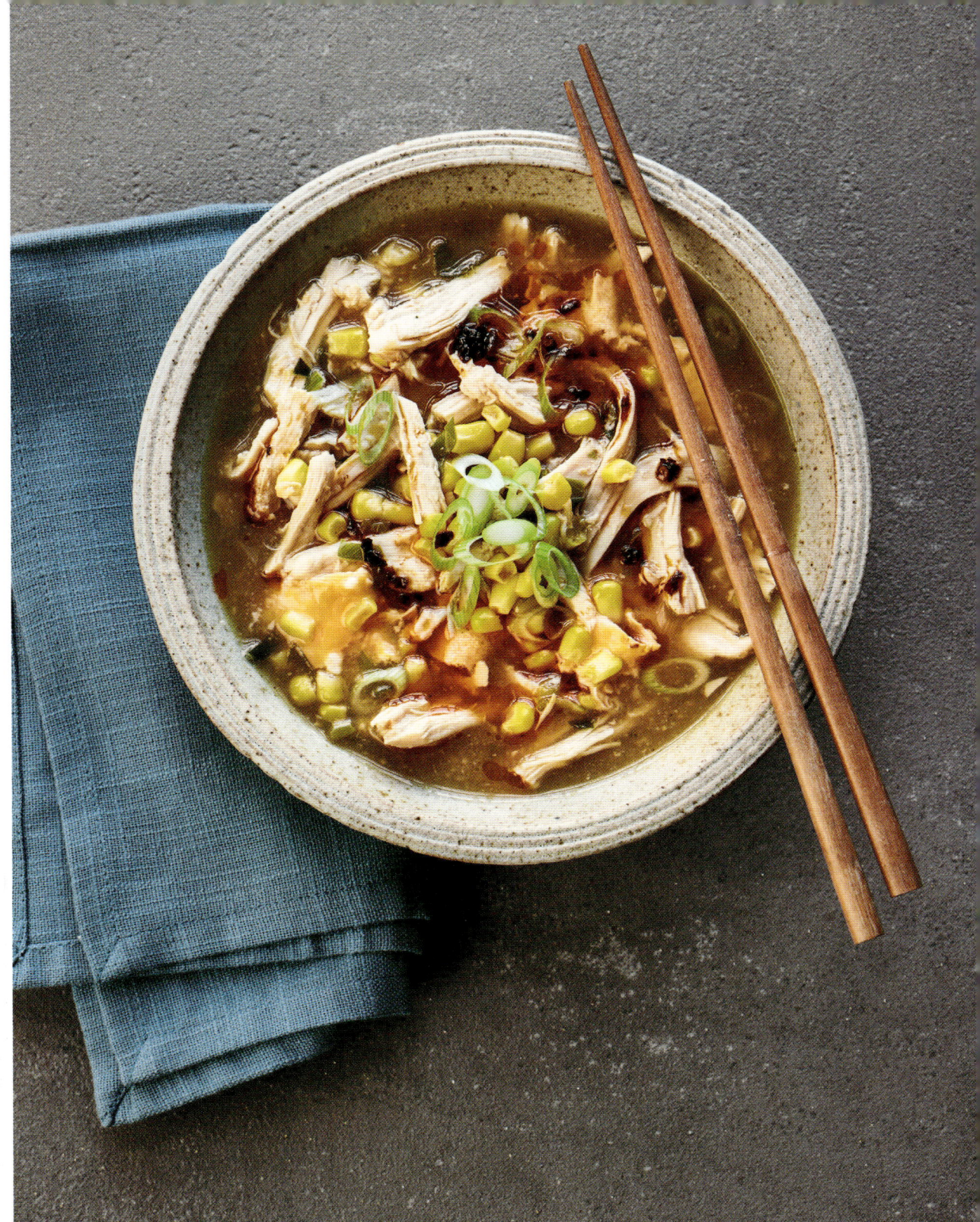

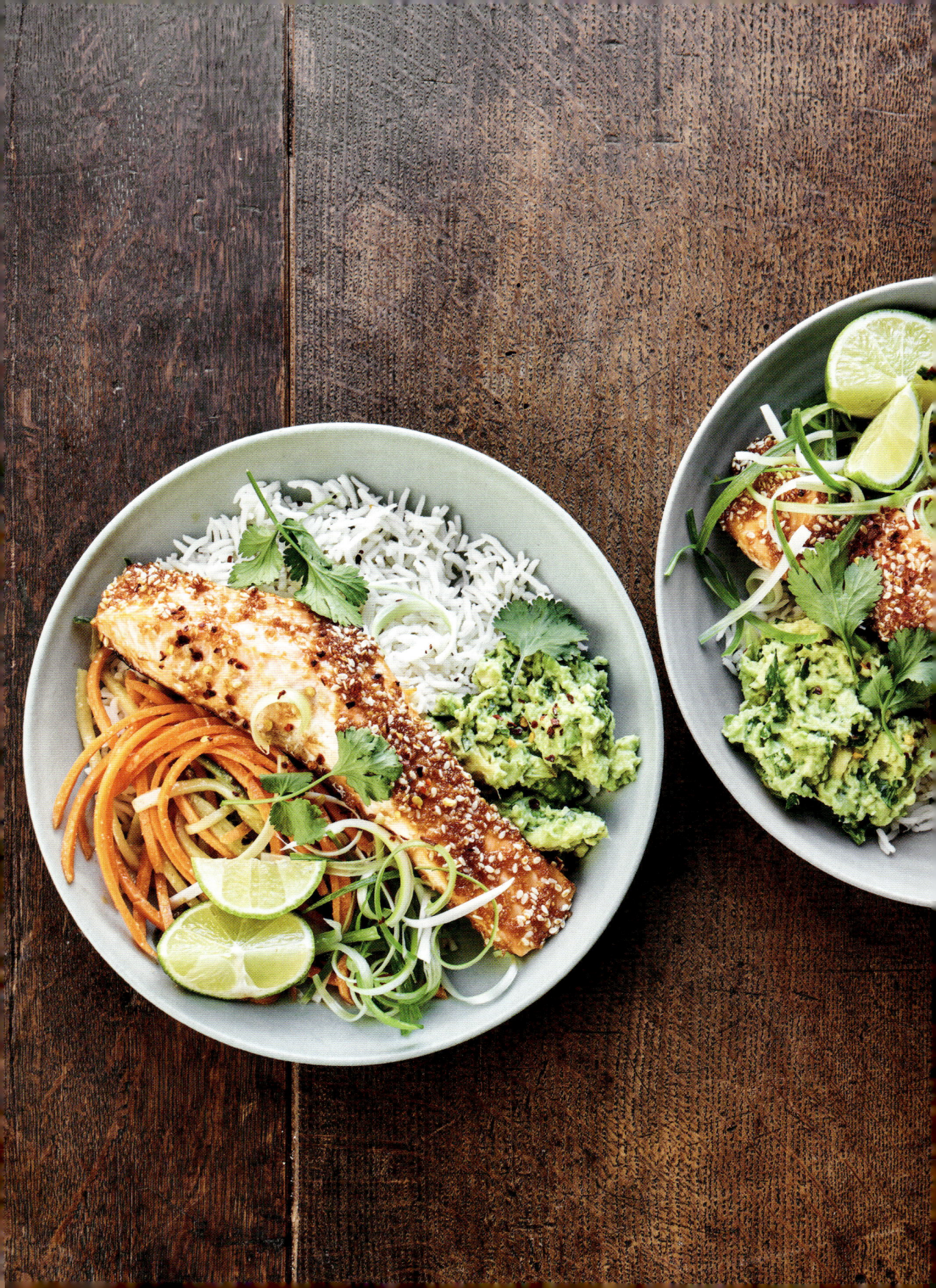

*A quick, easy rice bowl meal that is packed full of nutrition and ready in 15 minutes. It holds really well, and is perfect for lunch the next day. High in skin-supporting fats and vitamins C and E, this bowl is designed to support a glow from the inside out. Make it plant-based by simply swapping the fish for tofu.*

# Speedy Glow Wellness Bowls with Sticky Peanut Carrot Slaw

**SERVES 2**
**Under 640kcal,**
**28g protein per serving**

2 trout or salmon fillets
   (or any protein you like)
1 teaspoon garlic granules
1 teaspoon honey
Pinch of dried chilli flakes
1 teaspoon sesame seeds
1 medium ripe avocado,
   peeled and pitted
1 tablespoon chopped
   coriander (cilantro)
   or parsley
Zest and juice of 1 lime
250g (2 cups) cooked,
   seasoned rice
Salt and pepper

**FOR THE SLAW**
1 heaped teaspoon
   peanut butter
1 tablespoon rice vinegar
1 teaspoon garlic paste
1 scant teaspoon honey
1 tablespoon light soy sauce
1 carrot, julienned
¼ cucumber, deseeded
   and julienned
2 spring onions (scallions),
   julienned

Preheat the oven to 220°C/200°C fan (425°F) Gas Mark 7, or the air fryer to 190°C (375°F).

In a bowl, mix together the peanut butter, vinegar, garlic paste, honey and soy sauce. Add the carrot, cucumber and spring onions, mix to combine and leave to marinate.

Place the fish fillets in an oven dish and season with the garlic granules, honey, chilli flakes, sesame seeds and a pinch each of salt and pepper. Bake in the oven or air fryer for 7–10 minutes, until just cooked through.

In a bowl, chunkily mash the avocado with the chopped herbs, half the lime juice, and some of the zest. Season with salt and pepper.

Serve a base of warm rice. Top with the baked fish, slaw and a dollop of avocado.

*This aromatic but quick lunch is both filling and light, and will help you to avoid the afternoon slump. Add your vegetables and gyoza to the coconut soup base and simmer until cooked. You can use whatever vegetables you have at home, and it's ready in under 10 minutes – ideal for when you have back-to-back meetings.*

# Thai Red Coconut Gyoza Soup

**SERVES 1**
**Under 435kcal,**
**10g protein per serving**
**(for chicken gyoza)**

1 tablespoon Thai red
   curry paste

1–2 tablespoons light soy
   sauce, plus extra if needed

1 teaspoon ginger paste

150ml (⅔ cup) coconut
   milk (light or full fat)

150ml (⅔ cup) water

1 tablespoon fish sauce

6 gyoza (choose your
   favourite flavour)

1 small carrot, peeled
   and julienned

A few spears of Tenderstem
   broccoli cut into
   bite-sized pieces

½ red (bell) pepper,
   deseeded and sliced

1 large spring onion
   (scallion), sliced

1 teaspoon crispy chilli oil,
   to serve (optional)

In a deep pan, combine the curry paste, soy sauce, ginger paste, coconut milk and water. Bring to a gentle simmer, season with the fish sauce and simmer for 5 minutes.

Add the gyoza, carrot, broccoli, red pepper and spring onion (reserving some to garnish). Simmer until the gyoza are cooked and the vegetables are tender but still vibrant and crisp, about 5–7 minutes. Taste and season with more soy sauce if needed.

Pour into a serving bowl, drizzle with crispy chilli oil if desired, and garnish with the reserved spring onion.

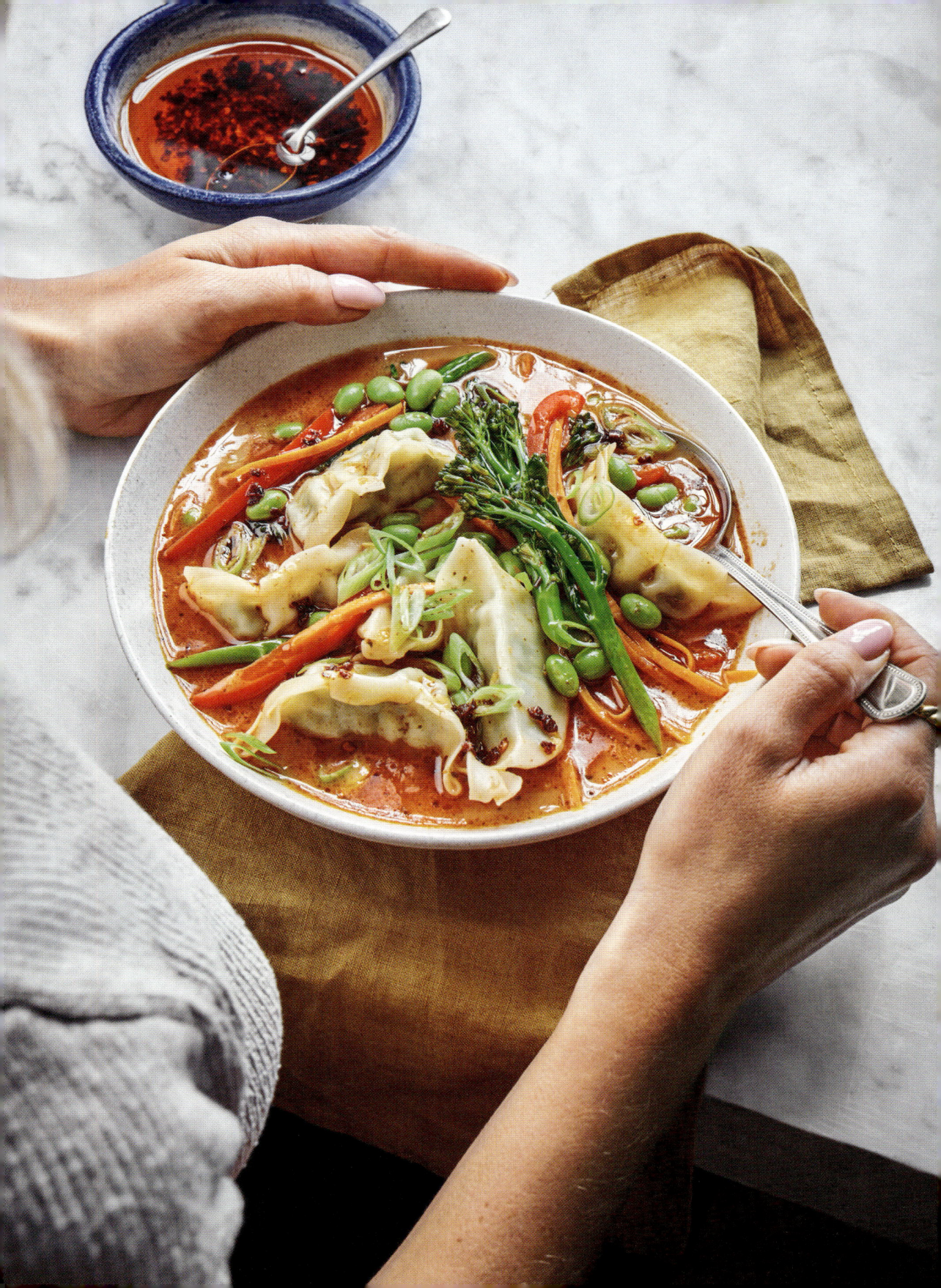

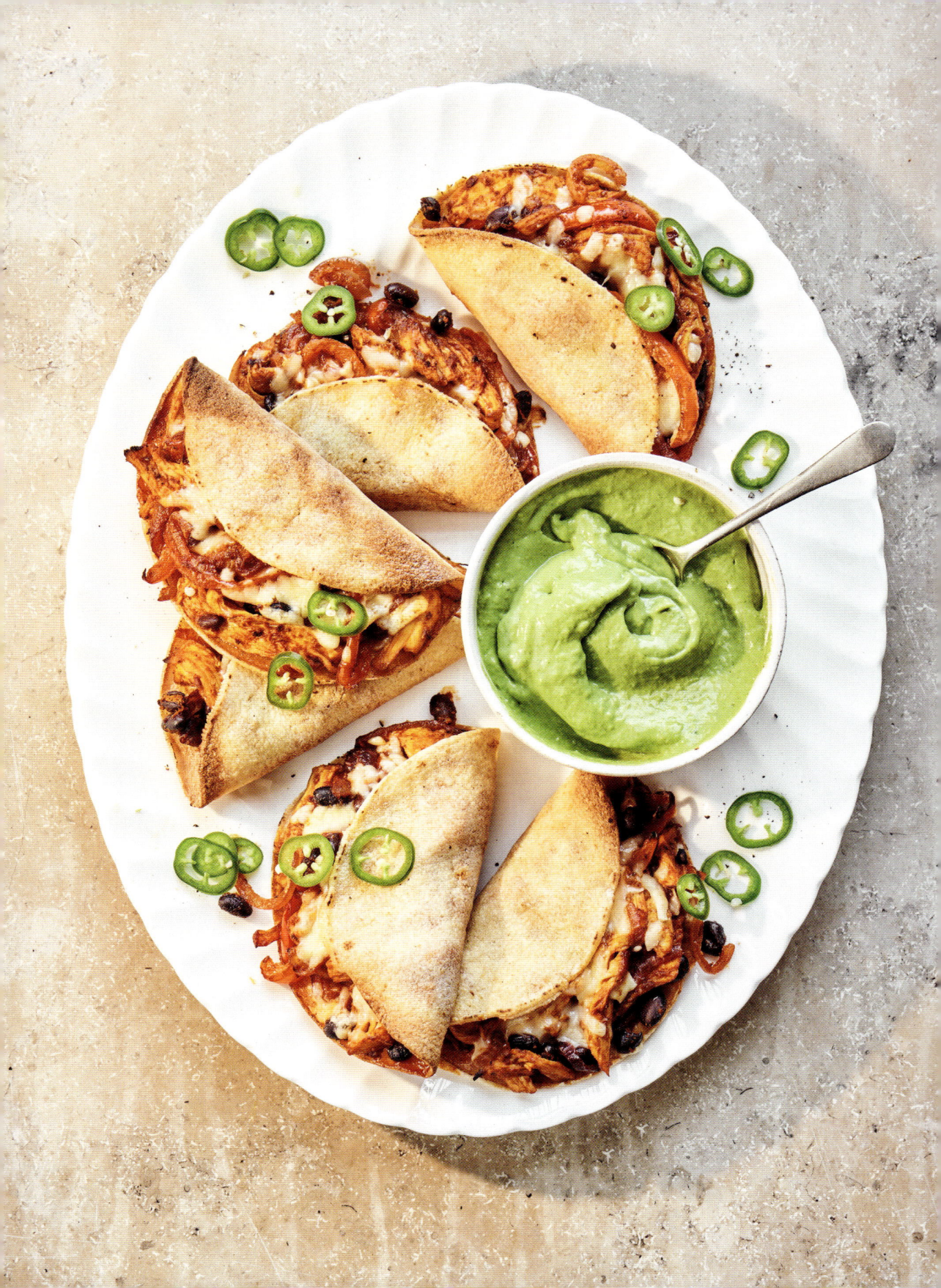

*These crispy baked chicken tacos are incredibly moreish. A spiced pulled chicken mix is stuffed into a corn tortilla with sharp Cheddar and baked until crisp and golden. Served with a creamy and tangy avocado sauce, these tacos are a joy to eat.*

# Crispy Baked Chicken Tacos

**SERVES 2**
**Under 600kcal,**
**40g protein per serving**

Olive oil, for cooking
    and brushing
1 red onion, finely sliced
1 red (bell) pepper, cored,
    deseeded and finely sliced
80g (2¾oz) cooked black
    beans (from a can)
1 teaspoon smoked paprika
½ teaspoon garlic granules
1 tablespoon chipotle paste
1 tablespoon tomato
    purée (paste)
2 tablespoons water
200g (7oz) cooked chicken
    breast, shredded
4 small corn (or
    wheat) tortillas
40g (1½oz) Cheddar
    cheese, grated
Salt and pepper
Sliced jalapeños or chillies,
    to garnish (optional)

**FOR THE AVOCADO SAUCE**
½ ripe avocado, peeled
    and pitted
2 heaped tablespoons Greek
    yogurt (0% or full fat)
1 spring onion (scallion),
    chopped
2 tablespoons jalapeños
    from a jar
Juice of 1 lime
Handful of coriander (cilantro)
    or parsley leaves
2 teaspoons honey

Preheat the oven to 230°C/210°C fan (450°F) Gas Mark 8, or the air fryer to 200°C (400°F).

Heat a little oil in a pan, add the red onion and pepper with a pinch of salt and sauté for about 5 minutes, until softened. Add in the black beans, smoked paprika, garlic granules, chipotle paste and tomato purée. Mix and add the water and shredded chicken. Sauté for another 3–4 minutes until the mixture is dry but still unctuous. Season to taste and set aside.

Put the avocado sauce ingredients in a blender or food processor and blend, seasoning to taste.

Brush or spray the tortillas with a little oil on one side. Flip and place some grated Cheddar on one half, then spoon in some of the chicken mix and fold in half.

If baking in the oven, place the filled tacos on a baking tray and bake for 6 minutes, then flip and bake for another 5 minutes. If not crisp, repeat for another 2–3 minutes on either side; they will crisp as they cool.

If using the air fryer, bake for 5 minutes, then flip and bake for another 5 minutes. If not crisp, repeat for another 2–3 minutes on either side; they will crisp as they cool.

Serve the crispy baked chicken tacos with the creamy avocado sauce, with extra sliced jalapeños or chillies to garnish, as desired.

*This refreshing and nutritious salad is perfect for a light and satisfying lunch. Served cold, it combines egg noodles with fresh vegetables and a flavourful tahini-soy dressing. It's also great for office lunches.*

# Sesame Soy Noodle Salad with Shredded Chicken

**SERVES 2**
**Under 645kcal,**
**44g protein per serving**

2 egg noodle nests
½ cucumber, julienned
1 large carrot, julienned
2 spring onions (scallions), finely sliced
½ red (bell) pepper, deseeded and thinly sliced
100g (3½oz) cooked edamame beans or peas
Handful of coriander (cilantro) leaves, chopped
200g (7oz) cooked chicken breast, shredded, or any protein of choice

**FOR THE DRESSING**
1 tablespoon tahini
1 tablespoon toasted sesame oil
1 tablespoon honey
Juice of 1 lime
2 tablespoons light soy sauce
1 tablespoon rice vinegar
1 teaspoon ginger paste
1 teaspoon garlic paste

Cook the noodles in a pan of salted boiling water, according to the packet instructions. Drain, saving a cup of the cooking water, then rinse under cold water to cool. Set aside.

In a large bowl, combine the cucumber, carrot, spring onions, red pepper, edamame, coriander and shredded chicken breast.

In a small bowl, whisk together the dressing ingredients until smooth.

Add the cooled noodles to the vegetable and chicken mixture. Pour the dressing over the top and toss everything together until well combined. Loosen with some of the reserved cooking water if needed. Serve immediately or refrigerate for up to 2 hours to allow the flavours to meld.

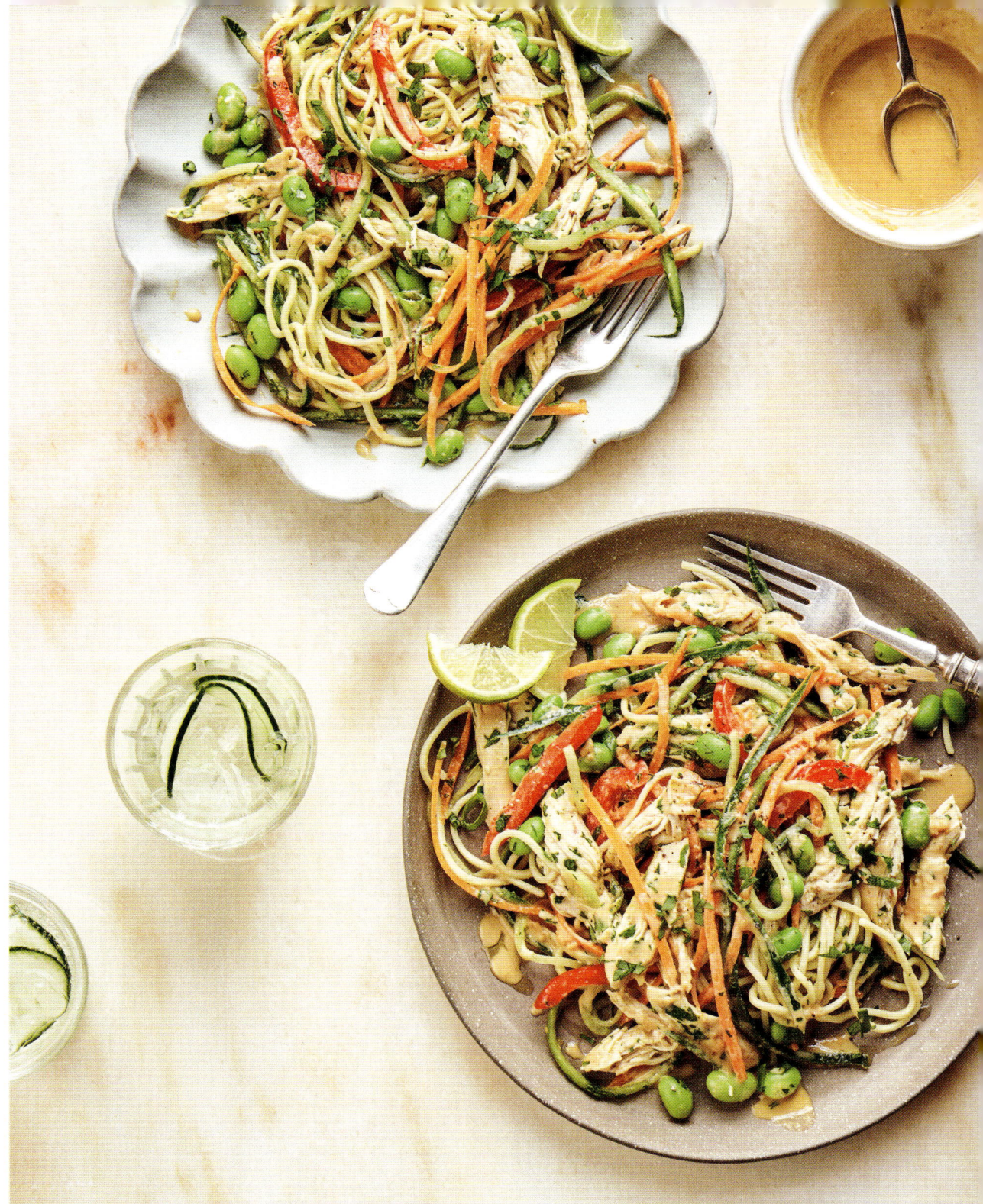

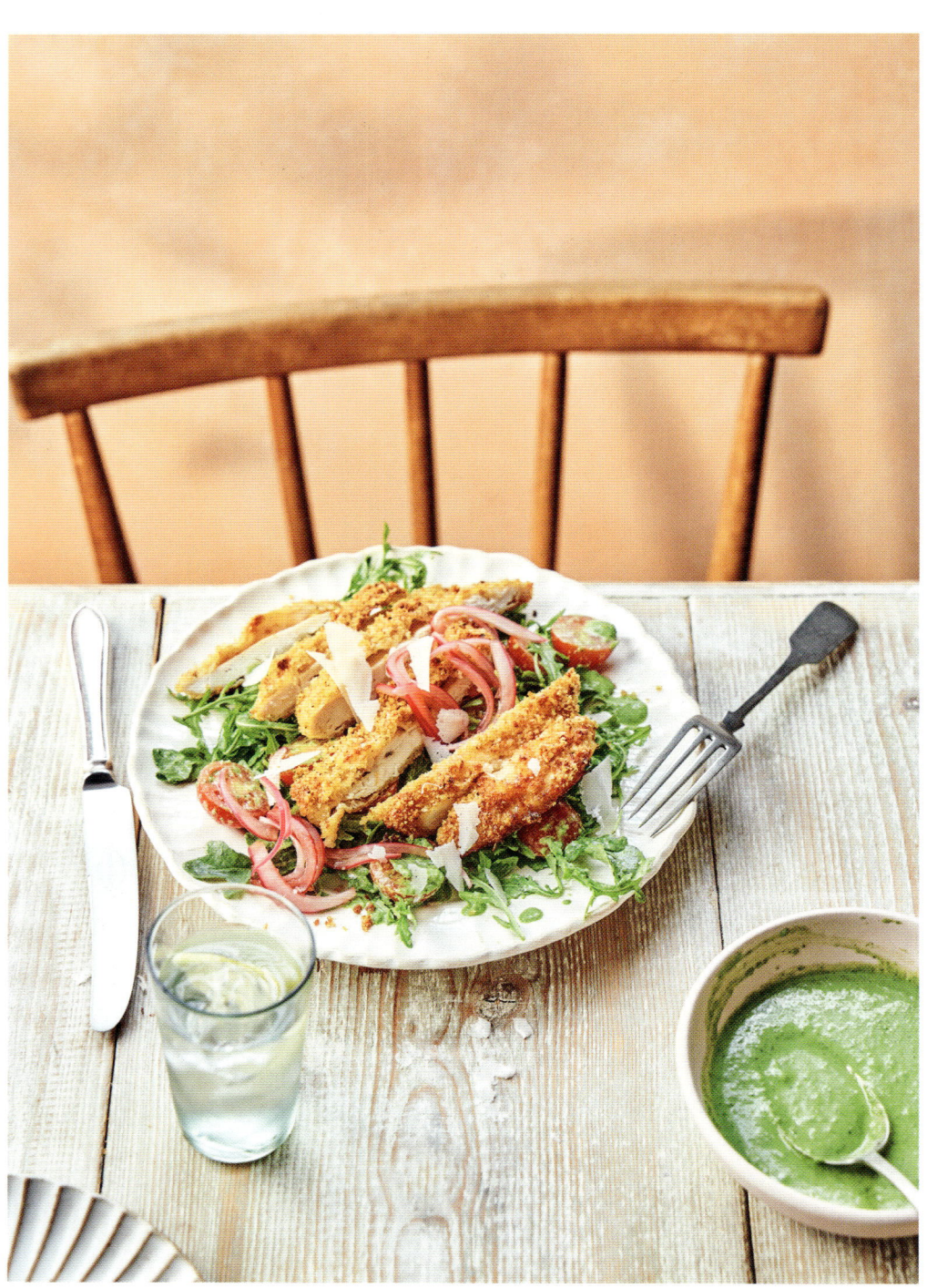

*The combination of the crispy Parmesan coating on this baked chicken with the bright pickled red onions and summer tomatoes tossed through a basil dressing is just a winner. This is a meal I could eat on repeat: perfectly balanced, high in protein and all the gorgeous plant diversity we want, while still tasting so good.*

# Crispy Baked Parmesan Chicken with Basil Goddess Salad

**SERVES 2**
**Under 430kcal,**
**52g protein per serving**

2 boneless, skinless chicken breasts

2 thick slices of stale bread (I use sourdough, but you can also use panko)

1 teaspoon garlic granules

½ teaspoon dried Italian herbs

15g (½oz) Parmesan cheese, grated

1 medium free-range egg, beaten

Cornflour (cornstarch) or plain (all-purpose) flour, for dredging

Olive oil, for cooking

Salt and pepper

**FOR THE PICKLE**

½ red onion

75ml (5 tablespoons) white wine vinegar

1 teaspoon honey

**FOR THE SALAD**

A few handfuls of cherry tomatoes, halved

A few handfuls of rocket (arugula)

30g (1oz) basil leaves

Juice of ½ lemon

2 tablespoons Greek yogurt (0% or full fat)

½ teaspoon garlic granules

10g (¼oz) Parmesan cheese, grated, plus extra to serve

Handful of chives, roughly chopped

1 teaspoon honey

Preheat the oven to 200°C/180°C fan (400°F) Gas Mark 6, or the air fryer to 200°C (400°F).

Butterfly the chicken breasts by placing your hand on top of one. Use a sharp knife to slice horizontally into the thicker part, being careful not to cut all the way through. Open it up to resemble a butterfly and season with salt and pepper.

Tear the stale bread into chunks and add to a food processor with the garlic granules, dried herbs, Parmesan and salt and pepper to taste. Process until fine, then transfer to a shallow bowl.

Place the beaten egg in another shallow bowl and the flour in a third bowl. Dredge each of the chicken breasts in flour, dip in the beaten egg, and press into the breadcrumb mixture. Repeat for a thicker crumb. Lightly drizzle with olive oil and cook in the oven for 20–25 minutes, or the air fryer for 20 minutes, until cooked and golden. Rest for 5 minutes before serving, ideally on a wire rack.

While the chicken cooks, in a small bowl, pickle the red onion in the vinegar and honey. Let sit while you prepare the salad and dressing.

Combine the halved cherry tomatoes and rocket in a large bowl.

Place the basil, lemon juice, yogurt, garlic granules, Parmesan, chives, honey and a good pinch each of salt and pepper in a blender and blend until smooth. Adjust the seasoning if needed with more lemon, honey, salt and pepper.

Toss the salad with the dressing and the pickled onions. Place on top of the chicken and serve with extra grated Parmesan.

*I love a good Greek salad, and I don't believe we should mess with the classics. This, however, is a version that makes it even better. Smashing the cucumber allows all the lovely dressing and feta to get into the cracks. Every bite is so full of flavour. Pair with any protein you like or serve as the perfect side.*

# Smashed Cucumber Greek Salad

**SERVES 4**
**Under 238kcal,**
**8g protein per serving**

1 cucumber

200g (7oz) feta cheese

1 tablespoon wholegrain mustard

Juice of 1 lemon

1 tablespoon extra virgin olive oil, plus extra (optional) to finish

Pinch of dried oregano, plus extra (optional) to finish

1 teaspoon honey

1 red onion, finely sliced

1 green (bell) pepper, deseeded and cut into thin strips

4 vine tomatoes, quartered

Handful of Kalamata olives, to taste

1 tablespoon capers

Quarter the cucumber lengthways, then smash each quarter lightly with the flat side of a knife or a rolling pin. Chop the cucumber into chunks. Place in a colander and leave to drain for a few minutes.

Crumble a third of the feta into a large mixing bowl and add the mustard, lemon juice, oil, oregano and honey. Mix well to combine into a creamy dressing.

Add the smashed cucumber, onion, pepper, tomatoes, olives and capers to the bowl with the dressing. Toss everything together to ensure the vegetables are well coated.

Crumble the remaining feta over the top of the salad, then gently toss again to distribute the feta without breaking it up too much.

Transfer the salad to a serving dish. If you like, finish with an extra sprinkle of oregano and/or drizzle of olive oil.

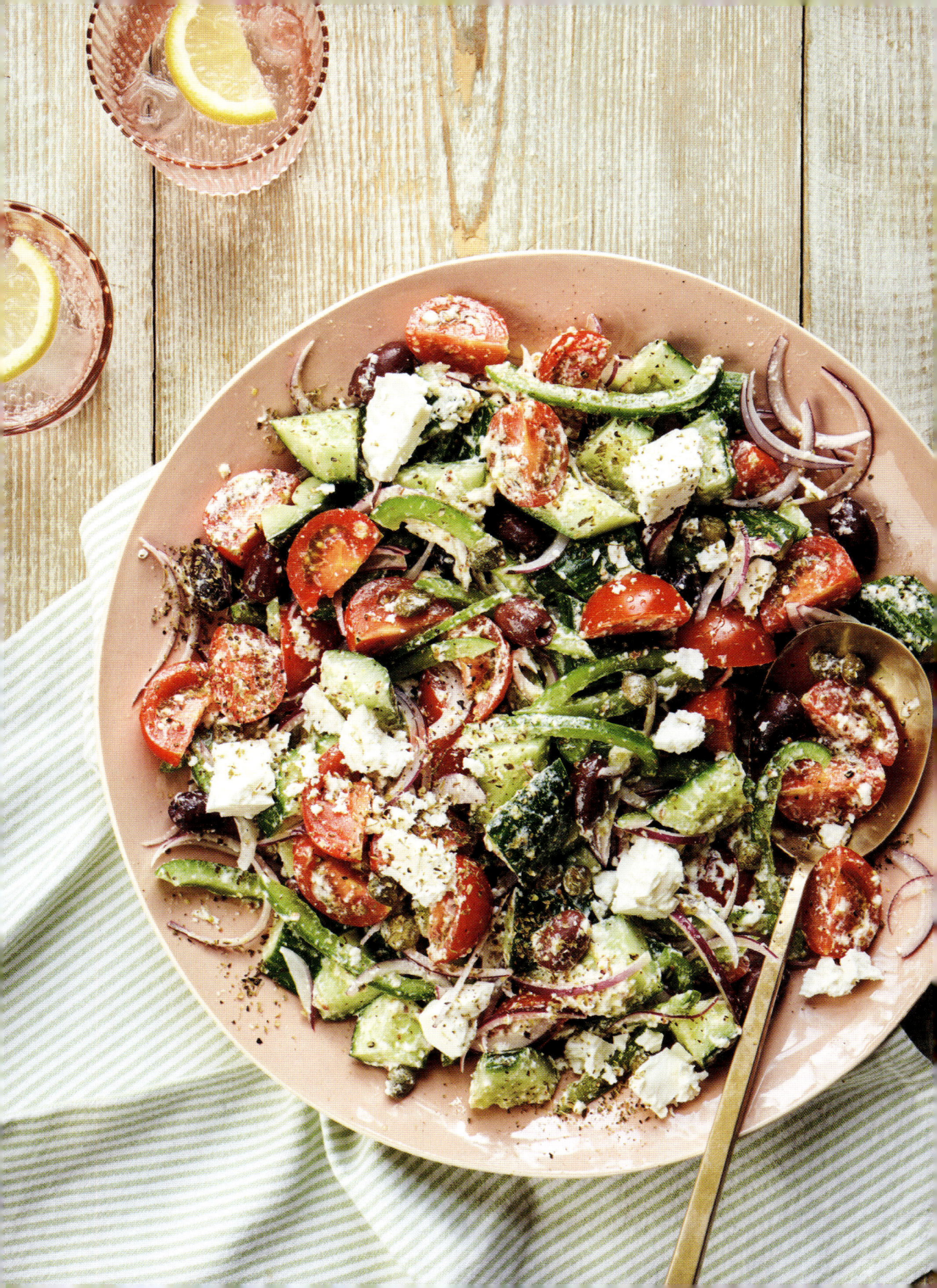

# Snacks

Butter Bean and Jalapeño Hummus | *Muhammara* | Sun-dried Tomato Tapenade | *High-protein Baked Artichoke Dip* | Savoury Granola Bars with Parmesan, Rosemary and Green Olives | *Soy and Honey Toasted Toppers* | Smoked Salmon Hand Rolls | *Spanakopita Filo Triangles* | Snacking Tuna Tostadas | *Classic Dill Pickles* | Spicy Pickled Carrots | *Sweet and Sour Pickled Red Onions*

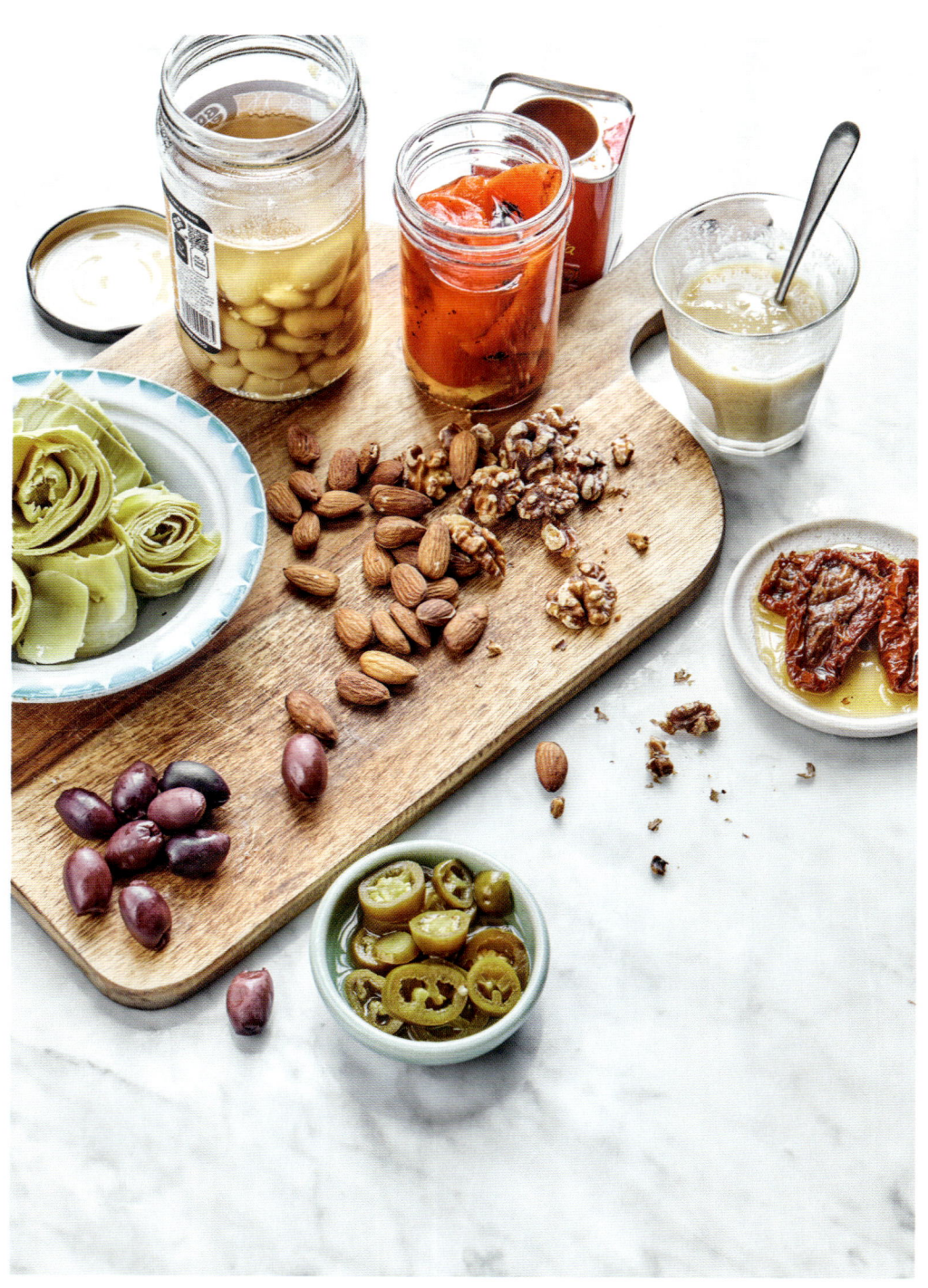

*Here is a creamy, spicy twist on the classic hummus. High in protein and fibre, it's perfect for dipping vegetables, spreading on toast or adding to your favourite wraps. This version uses butter beans for extra creaminess, and jalapeños from a jar for a mild kick.*

# Butter Bean and Jalapeño Hummus

**SERVES 4**
**Under 185kcal,**
**9g protein per serving**

400g (14oz) can of butter beans, drained and rinsed

2 tablespoons tahini

2 tablespoons lemon juice

1 tablespoon extra virgin olive oil

1–2 tablespoons (to taste) jalapeños from a jar, chopped

1 garlic clove, minced

¼ teaspoon ground cumin

¼ teaspoon smoked paprika

¼ teaspoon salt

60ml (¼ cup) water

In a food processor, combine all the ingredients except the water.

Blend until the mixture is smooth, slowly adding the water as needed to reach your desired consistency (you may need a little more).

Taste and adjust the seasoning or add more jalapeños if you prefer more heat. Serve immediately or store in an airtight container in the refrigerator for up to 5 days.

*This vibrant dish is a Middle Eastern red pepper and walnut dip. Rich in flavour and packed with healthy fats, it's perfect for dipping or spreading. My lighter version retains all the deliciousness with a few healthy tweaks.*

# Muhammara

**SERVES 4**
**Under 177kcal,**
**2g protein per serving**

---

3 large roasted red (bell)
  peppers from a jar, drained
1 tablespoon extra
  virgin olive oil
50g (scant ½ cup)
  walnuts, toasted
2 tablespoons breadcrumbs
  (wholegrain if possible)
1 garlic clove, minced
2 tablespoons pomegranate
  molasses
1 teaspoon ground cumin
½ teaspoon smoked paprika
¼ teaspoon salt
1–2 tablespoons lemon juice

In a food processor, combine all the ingredients and blend until smooth. If too thick, add a little water or more lemon juice to achieve the desired consistency.

Serve immediately or store in an airtight container in the refrigerator for up to 5 days.

*I can't claim this recipe as I owe my lovely friend Helene for this highly addictive tapenade. Deliciously tangy and savoury and packed with healthy fats, it's perfect for spreading, dipping or adding to your favourite dishes.*

# Sun-dried Tomato Tapenade

**SERVES 4**
**Under 290kcal,**
**3g protein per serving**

65g (2⅓ oz) sun-dried tomatoes

1 garlic clove, minced

75g (2⅔ oz) pitted Kalamata olives

50g (scant ½ cup) whole almonds, roasted

2–3 sprigs of rosemary, leaves only

1 tablespoon balsamic vinegar

4 tablespoons extra virgin olive oil

1 anchovy fillet in oil

Dried chilli flakes, to taste

Pinch of salt

1 teaspoon honey

Combine all the ingredients in a food processor and blend until smooth but still with texture, scraping down the sides as necessary. Taste and adjust the seasoning if necessary.

Serve immediately or store in an airtight container in the refrigerator for up to 5 days.

*Artichokes are full of prebiotic fibre, which means they help support and nourish the microbiome; this dip also sneaks in some extra protein while being creamy, cheesy and perfectly moreish.*

# High-protein Baked Artichoke Dip

**SERVES 8**
**Under 100kcal,**
**7g protein per serving**

200g (scant 1 cup) full-fat cottage cheese

150g (⅔ cup) light cream cheese, softened

60g (2¼oz) Parmesan cheese, grated, plus extra for topping

1 large garlic clove, minced

1 banana shallot, finely diced

½ teaspoon each of salt and pepper

1 tablespoon chopped chives

150g (5½oz) frozen chopped spinach, defrosted and excess water squeezed out

400g (14oz) can of artichoke hearts in water, drained and chopped

Pinch of dried chilli flakes

Preheat the oven to 200°C/180°C fan (400°F) Gas Mark 6.

Add the cottage cheese and cream cheese to a blender and blend until smooth, but don't over-blend. Add the Parmesan, garlic, shallot, salt and pepper and blend once more.

Fold in the chopped chives, spinach, artichoke hearts and chilli flakes until evenly distributed. Transfer the mixture to a baking dish, spread it out evenly and bake in the oven for 25–30 minutes or until hot and bubbly. If you like a crispy top, turn on the grill (broiler) setting for the last 3–5 minutes of baking, watching closely to avoid burning.

Remove from the oven and let cool slightly before serving with crudités, spread on toasts, or enjoy with crackers.

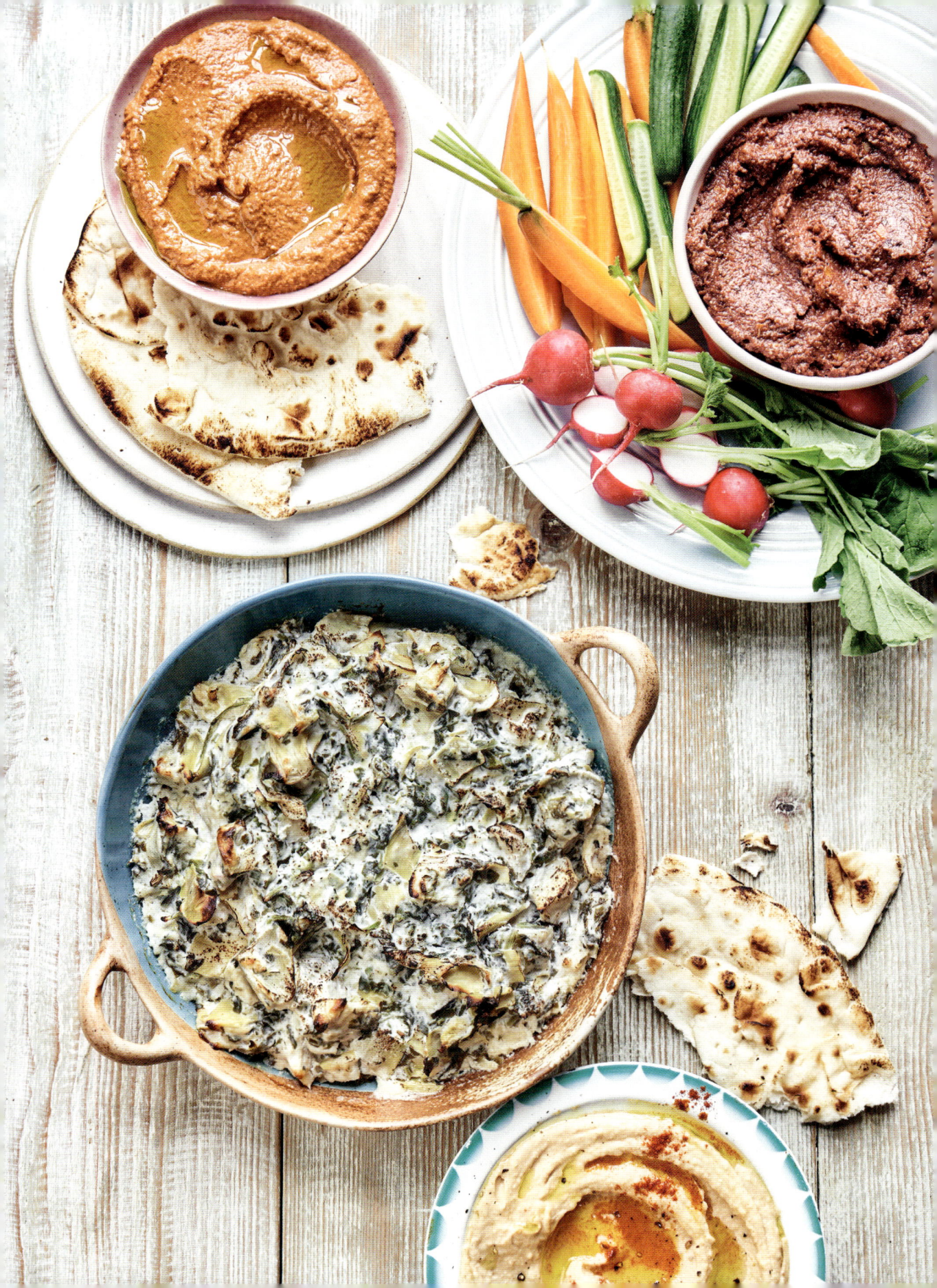

*These savoury granola bars are a brilliant twist on the traditional sweet version, packing in lots of plant protein, healthy fats and fibre. Full of the umami flavours of Parmesan, rosemary and green olives, they make for a perfect snack, and you can also adapt and swap around any of the flavours to suit you. To boost the protein content I have added some quinoa and chickpea flour.*

# Savoury Granola Bars with Parmesan, Rosemary and Green Olives

**MAKES 12 BARS**
**Under 210kcal,**
**8g protein per serving**

200g (1½ cups) rolled oats

100g (3½oz) cooked quinoa

50g (1¾oz) chickpea (gram) flour

100g (3½oz) Parmesan cheese, grated

50g (1¾oz) green olives, pitted and finely chopped

2 tablespoons rosemary leaves, finely chopped

50g (scant ½ cup) sunflower seeds

50g (scant ½ cup) pumpkin seeds

2 large free-range eggs

3 tablespoons olive oil

2 tablespoons honey

½ teaspoon each of salt and pepper

Preheat the oven to 200°C/180°C fan (400°F) Gas Mark 6. Line a 23 x 33cm (9 x 13 inch) baking tin (pan) with nonstick baking paper.

In a large bowl, combine the oats, quinoa, chickpea flour, Parmesan, olives, rosemary, sunflower and pumpkin seeds. Mix well to ensure even distribution.

In a separate bowl, beat together the eggs, olive oil and honey until well combined.

Pour the wet ingredients into the dry ingredients. Add the salt and pepper and mix thoroughly until all the ingredients are well combined.

Transfer the mixture to the prepared tin and press down firmly to ensure it is compact and evenly spread. Bake in the oven for 25–30 minutes or until the edges are golden brown and the centre is set.

Remove from the oven and allow to cool in the tin for about 10 minutes, then transfer to a wire rack to cool completely. Once cooled, cut into 12 bars and store in an airtight container at room temperature for up to a week.

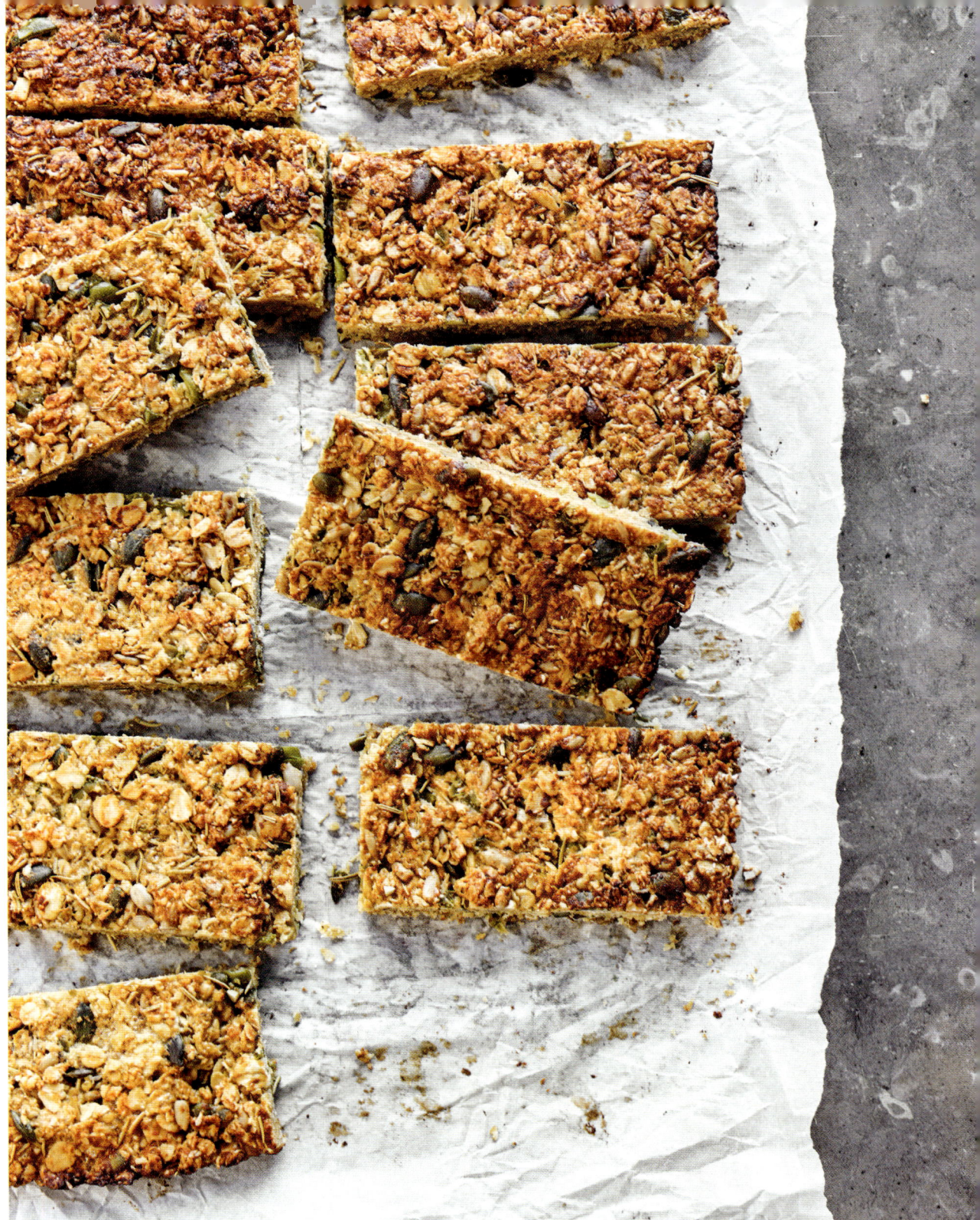

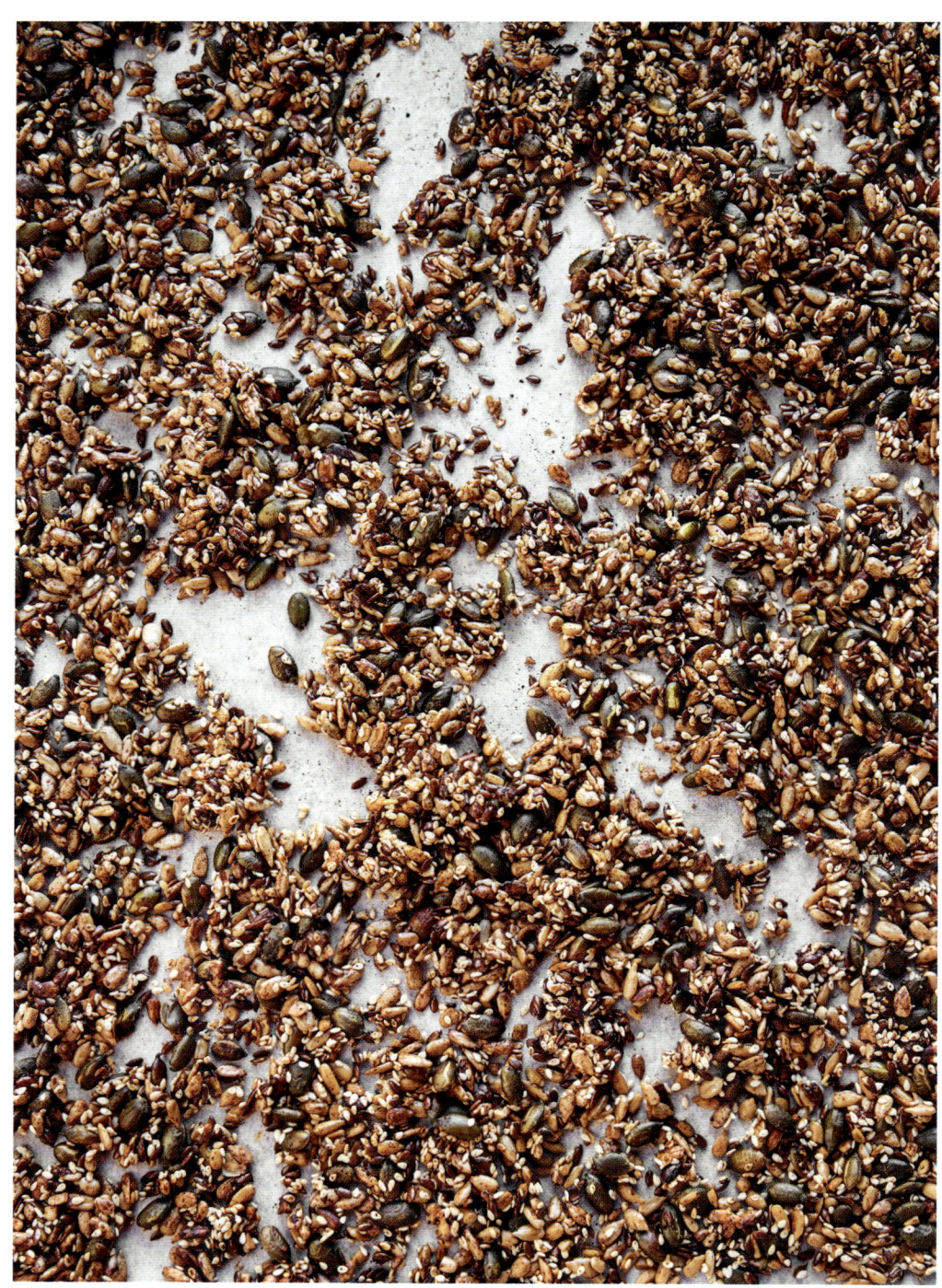

*This toasted seed mix is perfect for snacking on or scattering over your favourite dishes. With a balance of sweet and salty, it is seriously addictive. Enjoy a handful as a snack on its own, or scatter over salads or roasted vegetables for added flavour and crunch.*

# Soy and Honey Toasted Toppers

**MAKES ABOUT 250G (9OZ)**
**Under 150 kcal (per 25g),**
**6.4g protein (per 25g)**

250g (2 cups) mixed seeds
 (such as sunflower,
 pumpkin, etc.)
1 teaspoon olive oil
½ teaspoon garlic granules
1 tablespoon sesame seeds
¼ teaspoon salt
1 teaspoon light soy sauce
1 teaspoon honey
Pinch of cayenne pepper

Preheat the oven to 180°C/160°C fan (350°F) Gas Mark 4 and line a baking tray with nonstick baking paper.

In a large bowl, combine all the ingredients and mix well until all the seeds are evenly coated. Spread out in a single layer on the lined baking tray.

Bake in the oven for 10–15 minutes, stirring halfway through, until the seeds are golden brown and fragrant.

Remove from the oven and let cool completely on the baking tray. Once cooled, transfer to an airtight container for storage.

*These hand rolls are one of my favourite quick and healthy snack options. They have the flavours of sushi but just enough protein and spice to satisfy me. I use smoked salmon here, but you can swap it for any protein you like. You can also make them veggie by replacing the salmon with marinated tofu or chickpeas.*

# Smoked Salmon Hand Rolls

**MAKES 4**
**Under 110kcal,**
**8g protein per serving**

4 sheets of nori seaweed
4 heaped teaspoons
   light cream cheese
100g (3½oz) smoked
   salmon, sliced
½ cucumber, julienned
1 carrot, julienned
2 spring onions (scallions),
   finely sliced
Sriracha, to taste

Lay a sheet of nori on a flat surface, shiny side down.

Spread a heaped teaspoon of cream cheese evenly over the bottom half of the nori sheet. Arrange a quarter of the smoked salmon slices on top of the cream cheese. Add a small handful of cucumber, carrot and spring onion on top of the salmon.

Drizzle a small amount of sriracha over the vegetables and salmon. Starting from the bottom, carefully roll the nori sheet upwards, pressing gently to form a tight roll.

Repeat the process with the remaining nori sheets and ingredients to make 4 hand rolls. Slice each roll in half diagonally and serve immediately.

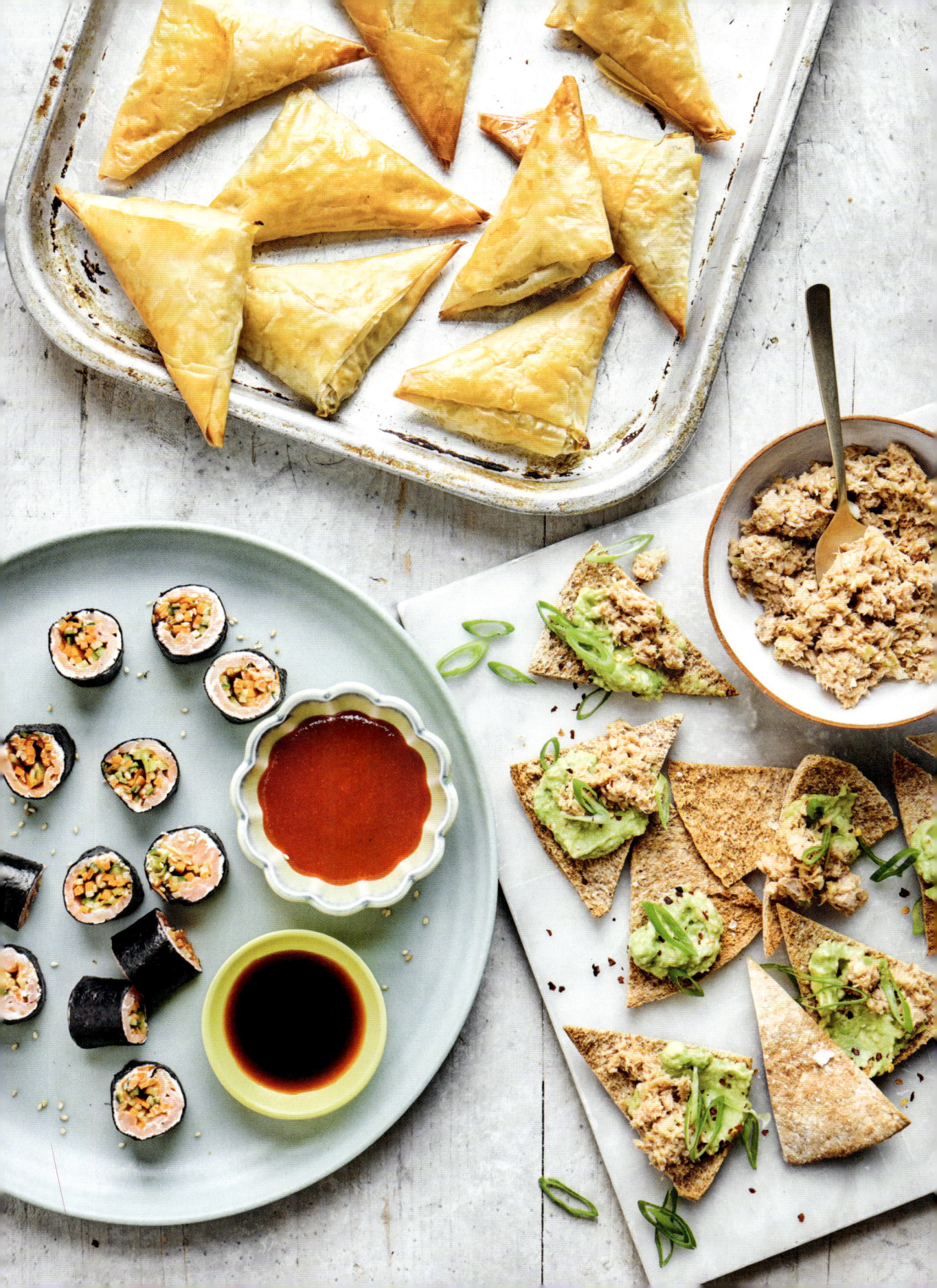

*These spinach, cottage cheese and feta bites are a healthier take on the traditional spanakopita; the deliciously tangy filling is packed with nutritious spinach.*

# Spanakopita Filo Triangles

**MAKES ABOUT 18**
**Under 65kcal,**
**3.5g protein per serving**

150g (5½oz) cottage cheese
100g (3½oz) feta
    cheese, crumbled
150g (5½oz) baby spinach
    leaves, wilted and chopped
2 spring onions
    (scallions), diced
1 tablespoon fresh dill
    and mint, chopped
1 medium free-range
    egg, beaten
250g (9oz) filo (phyllo) pastry
Olive oil spray
Salt and pepper

Preheat the oven to 180°C/160°C fan (350°F) Gas Mark 4.

In a bowl, combine the cottage cheese, feta, spinach, spring onions, dill, mint and egg. Season with salt and pepper to taste.

Place 1 sheet of filo pastry on a flat surface and lightly spray with olive oil. Top with a second pastry sheet to make 2 layers. Cut lengthways into 3 strips. Place 1 heaped teaspoon of the spinach and cheese mixture in the corner of the first layered pastry strip. Fold over diagonally to form a triangle. Continue folding, making roughly 4 or 5 folds while keeping the triangular shape. Discard any excess pastry.

Place the finished triangles on a lined baking tray. Prepare the next pastry strips in the same way until you have a total of 18 triangles. Spray the tops with olive oil.

Bake in the oven for 25–30 minutes or until golden and crisp. (Alternatively, air fry at 180°C/350°F for 10–12 minutes.) Serve immediately or store in an airtight container in the refrigerator for up to 4 days.

*These tuna tostadas are a delight, and once you start making them as a snack, I promise you will be addicted. Simple baked pitta crisps are topped with a sesame-soy tuna mix and creamy avocado, making for a perfect bite-size snack. You can make each component separately and store for the week.*

# Snacking Tuna Tostadas

**SERVES 4**
**Under 180kcal,**
**13g protein per serving**

150g (5½oz) can of tuna
  in water, drained
1 tablespoon light soy sauce
1 tablespoon sesame oil
1 teaspoon sesame seeds
2 spring onions (scallions),
  finely chopped, plus
  extra to finish
½ teaspoon ginger paste
2 heaped tablespoons Greek
  yogurt (0% or full fat)
1 small ripe avocado,
  peeled and pitted
Juice of ½ lime
Pinch of dried chilli flakes
½ teaspoon garlic granules
Salt and pepper

**FOR THE BAKED PITTA CRISPS**
2 wholemeal (wholewheat)
  pitta breads
Olive oil spray

Preheat the oven to 200°C/180°C fan (400°F) Gas Mark 6.

Cut the pitta breads into small triangles or circles, about 6 pieces per pitta. Arrange the pieces on a baking tray and lightly spray with olive oil and sprinkle with salt. Bake for 10–12 minutes or until golden and crispy, then remove from the oven and let cool slightly.

Meanwhile, prepare the tuna topping. In a bowl, mix the drained tuna, soy sauce, sesame oil, sesame seeds, spring onions, ginger paste and yogurt. Season with salt and pepper to taste.

Crush the avocado with salt, pepper, lime juice, chilli flakes and garlic granules. Top each slightly cooled pitta crisp with a spoonful of the avocado then the tuna mixture, and finish with an extra sprinkle of spring onion.

Store the pitta crisps in an airtight container and the tuna mix in the refrigerator to enjoy in the week.

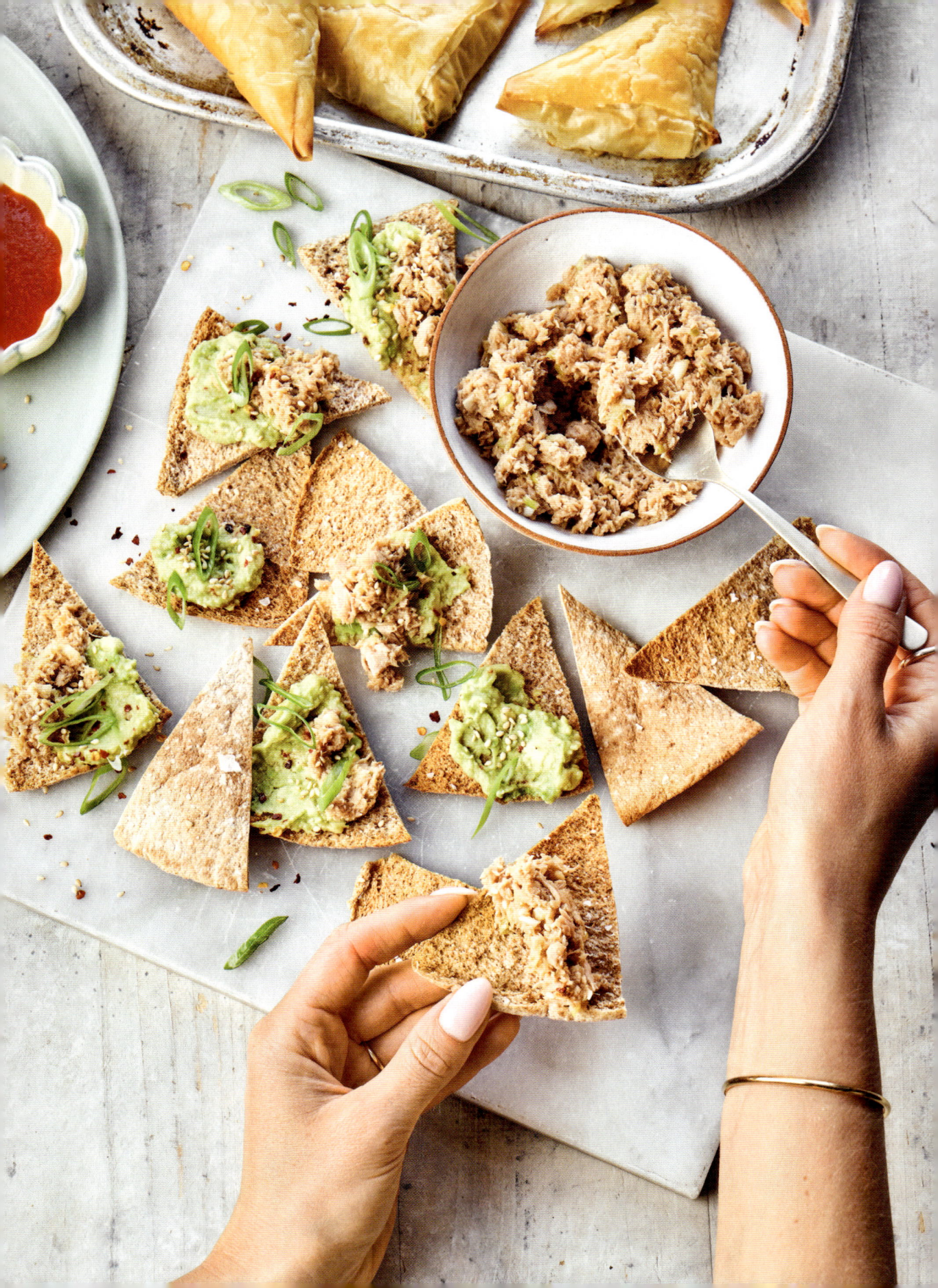

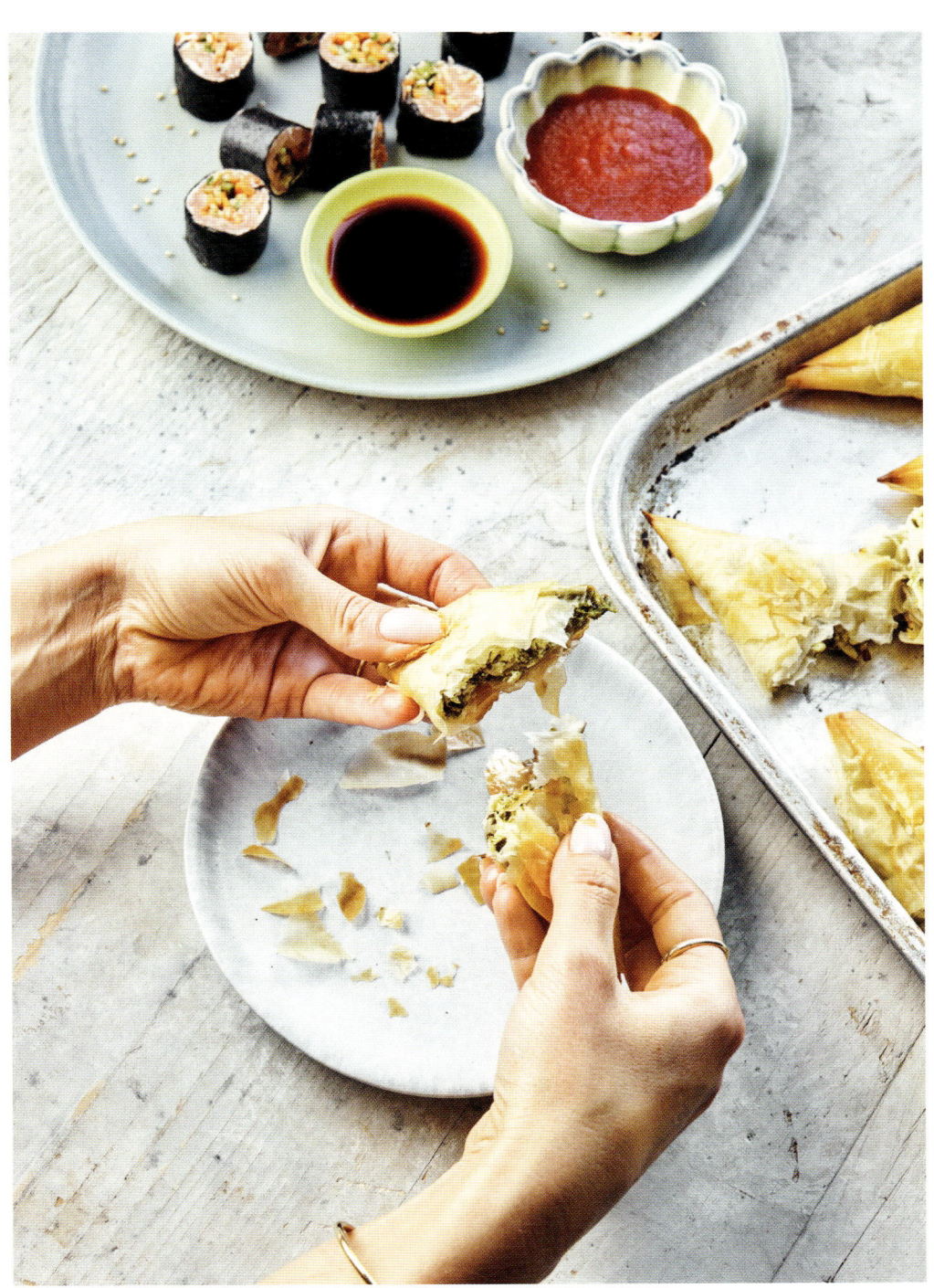

# Guide to Making Pickles

I love making my own pickles, which I always used to get my clients to do. Pickling is an ancient method of food preservation that not only extends the shelf life of vegetables but also enhances their flavours. This guide will help you master the basics of pickling with a simple ratio, and offers three different pickle recipes that you can use to prep and add to any dish. Not only are they delicious, they also have an amazing array of health-promoting benefits.

## HEALTH BENEFITS OF PICKLES

**Blood Sugar Balance:** The vinegar in pickles can help improve insulin sensitivity, which aids in regulating blood sugar levels. This is particularly beneficial for people with type 2 diabetes or those looking to manage their blood sugar.

**Satiety:** Pickles are light but full of flavour, making them a great addition to enhance satiety when eating a meal. The fibre content in pickled vegetables also contributes to a feeling of fullness, helping to regulate appetite.

**Gut Health:** Fermented pickles contain probiotics, beneficial bacteria that support a healthy gut microbiome. A balanced microbiome is crucial for digestion, nutrient absorption and overall immune function.

**Antioxidants:** Pickled vegetables retain many of their original nutrients, including antioxidants like vitamins C and E. Antioxidants help protect the body from oxidative stress and reduce inflammation.

## PICKLING RATIO

For a basic pickling brine, use the following ratio: 1 part vinegar (for acidity and preservation); 1 part water; 10% sugar (by weight of the total liquid).

Adjust the sugar content to your taste preference. You can also infuse the brine with various herbs, spices and aromatics to create unique mixes.

## BEST VEGETABLES TO PICKLE

Cucumbers | Carrots | Cauliflower | Green beans | Radishes | (Bell) peppers
Onions | Beetroot (beet) | Cabbage | Courgettes (zucchini)

# Pickle Recipes

## Classic Dill Pickles

**MAKES 1 JAR**
**Under 240kcal,**
**4g protein per serving**

240ml (1 cup) white vinegar
240ml (1 cup) water
30g (2½ tablespoons) sugar
15g (½oz) salt
2 garlic cloves, sliced
1 teaspoon mustard seeds
Handful of dill sprigs
400g (14oz) cucumber slices

Combine the vinegar, water, sugar and salt in a saucepan and bring to the boil.

Place the garlic, mustard seeds and fresh dill in a sterilised jar. Pack cucumber slices tightly into the jar.

Pour the hot brine over the cucumbers, leaving 1cm (½ inch) headroom.

Seal the jar and let it cool. Refrigerate for at least 24 hours before serving.

## Spicy Pickled Carrots

**MAKES 1 JAR**
**Under 332kcal,**
**2g protein per serving**

240ml (1 cup) white vinegar
240ml (1 cup) water
30g (2½ tablespoons) sugar
15g (½oz) salt
2 garlic cloves, sliced
1 teaspoon dried chilli flakes
1 teaspoon black peppercorns
400g (14oz) carrot sticks

Combine the vinegar, water, sugar and salt in a saucepan and bring to the boil.

Place the garlic, dried chilli flakes and black peppercorns in a sterilised jar. Pack the carrot sticks tightly into the jar.

Pour the hot brine over the carrots, leaving 1cm (½ inch) headroom.

Seal the jar and let it cool. Refrigerate for at least 24 hours before serving.

# Sweet and Sour Pickled Red Onions

**MAKES 1 JAR**
**Under 354kcal,**
**2g protein per serving**

240ml (1 cup) apple
  cider vinegar
240ml (1 cup) water
45g (¼ cup) sugar
15g (½oz) salt
1 teaspoon mustard seeds
3 large red onions,
  finely sliced

Combine the vinegar, water, sugar and salt in a saucepan and bring to the boil.

Place the mustard seeds in a sterilised jar. Pack the red onion slices tightly into the jar.

Pour the hot brine over the onions, leaving 1cm (½ inch) headroom.

Seal the jar and let it cool. Refrigerate for at least 24 hours before serving.

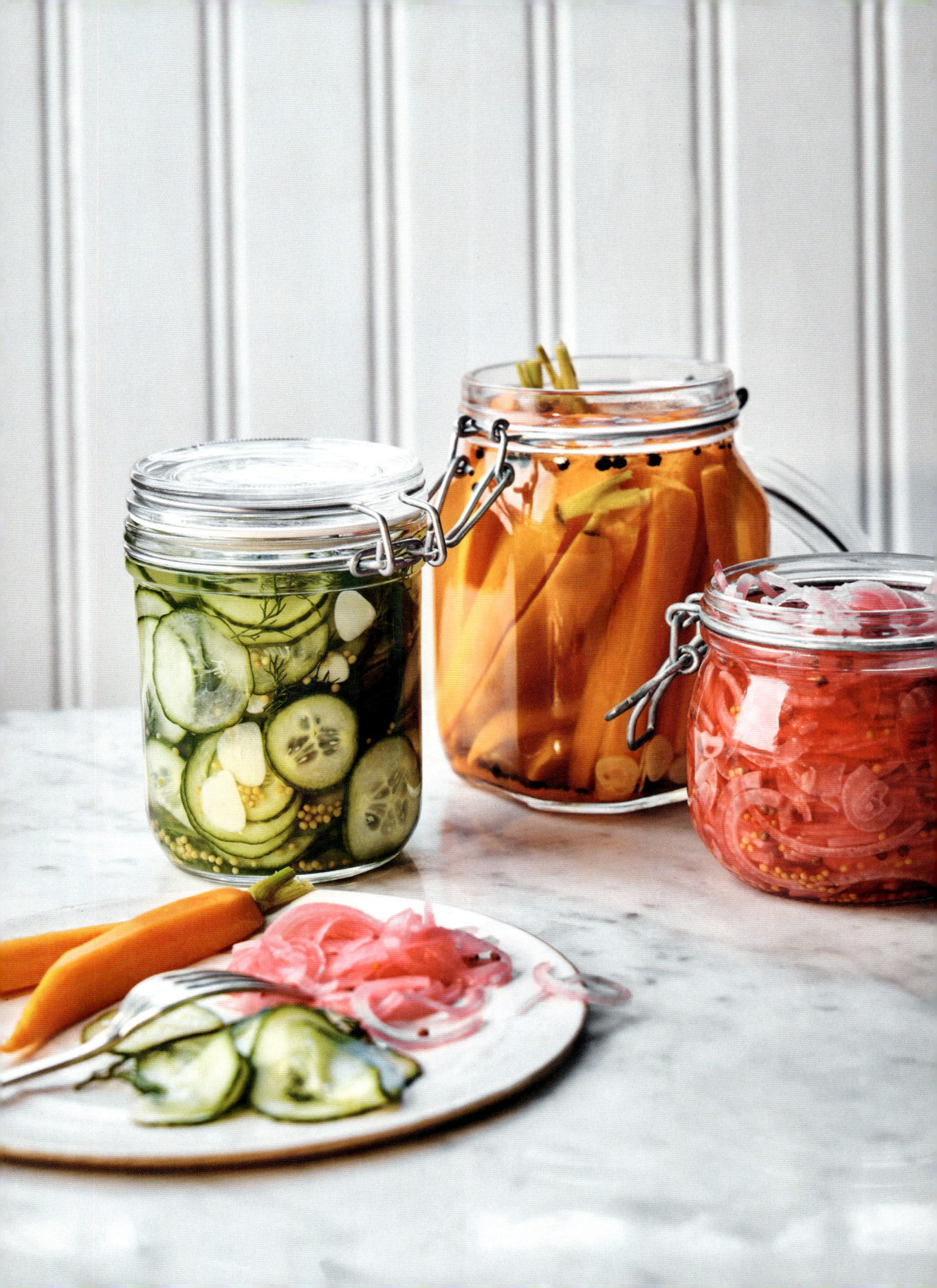

# Dinner

Whipped Ricotta and Slow-roasted Tomato Gnocchi | *Crab, Chilli and Courgette Spaghetti* | Baked Salmon with Sauce Vierge | *Yogurt Harissa Chicken with Smoky Rice* | Longevity Minestrone | *Jalapeño, Honey and Lime Marinade* | Yogurt Harissa Marinade | *Coconut and Lemongrass Marinade* | Aubergine Cannelloni with Garlic and Herb Crumb | *Loaded Harissa Chicken Potatoes with Herby Feta* | Crispy Potato Fish Pie Bake | *Lamb and Feta Burgers with Cucumber Slaw and Garlic Yogurt* | Simple Super Greens Pasta | *Smoky Mexican White Bean Chilli* | Pork and Caramelised Apple Meatballs | *Sticky Orange and Cashew Chicken Bowls* | Better-than-takeout Healthy Pad Thai | *Creamy Almond Butter Curry* | One-pan Pea, Parma Ham and Parmesan Gnocchi | *Easy One-pot Creamy Mushroom Risotto* | Seared Chipotle Steak Bowls with Charred Corn Salad | *Tikka Cod with Caramelised Onion Rice* | Prawn Saganaki Orzo | *Spatchcock Chicken with Rosemary Pesto* | Crushed Pipérade Potatoes with Garlic Yogurt and Sea Bass

*I love simple, quick, healthy meals, and this gnocchi is just that. Slow-roasting the tomatoes, garlic and aubergine creates a really intensely flavoured sauce that pairs so well with the creamy lemon and Parmesan ricotta. Add in any cooked protein with the gnocchi to make this more complete. Leftovers make the perfect lunch for the next day.*

# Whipped Ricotta and Slow-roasted Tomato Gnocchi

**SERVES 2**

**Under 375kcal,**

**12g protein per serving**

250g (9oz) cherry tomatoes

1 small aubergine (eggplant), cut into small cubes

12 pitted Kalamata olives, quartered

1 tablespoon capers

Pinch of chilli flakes

1 teaspoon dried oregano

1 tablespoon balsamic vinegar

2 garlic cloves, unpeeled, smashed

Olive oil, for drizzling

1 tablespoon tomato purée (paste)

4 tablespoons water

Handful of basil leaves, torn

250g (9oz) fresh gnocchi

Salt and pepper

**FOR THE WHIPPED RICOTTA**

2 generous tablespoons ricotta cheese

Zest of ½ lemon

20g (¾oz) Parmesan cheese, grated, plus extra to serve

Preheat the oven to 210°C/190°C fan (410°F) Gas Mark 6½.

In an ovenproof dish, combine the cherry tomatoes, aubergine, olives, capers, chilli flakes, oregano and vinegar, and season with salt and pepper. Add the garlic cloves and drizzle a little olive oil to evenly coat the vegetables.

Cover the dish with foil and bake in the oven for 25 minutes, then remove the foil and add the tomato purée and 2 tablespoons of the water, mix and bake for another 10 minutes until the tomatoes are collapsing and everything is soft. Remove the garlic, peel off the skin, mince the flesh and add it back to the sauce, along with the basil and remaining 2 tablespoons of water.

For the whipped ricotta, combine the ricotta, lemon zest, Parmesan and salt and pepper to taste.

Cook the gnocchi in a pan of salted boiling water, according to the packet instructions. Drain, saving a cup of the cooking water. Add the warm gnocchi to the sauce and mix. Loosen with the reserved gnocchi water, if needed, to make it more saucy.

Serve topped with a heaped tablespoon of ricotta and an extra grating of Parmesan.

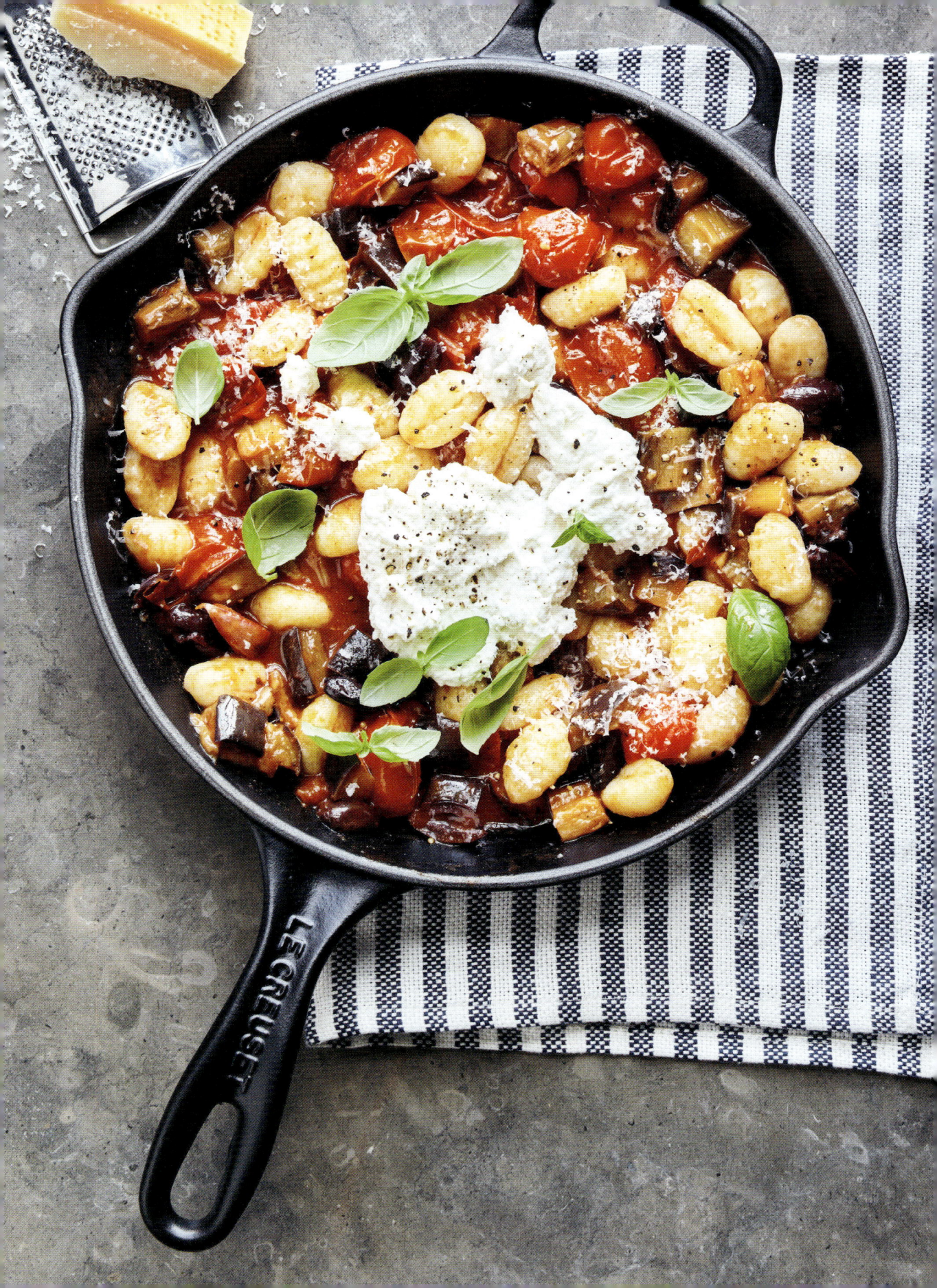

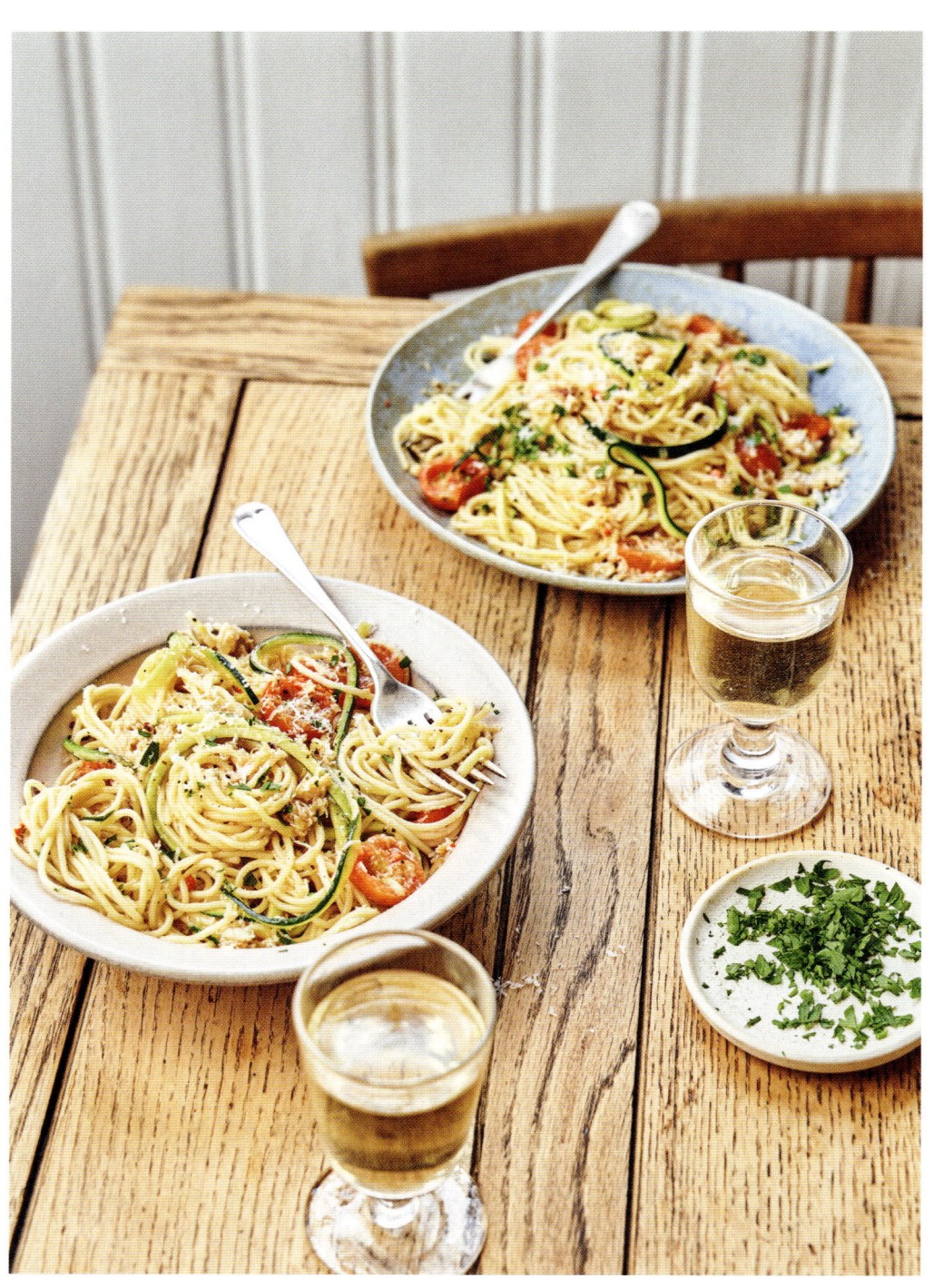

*My go-to date or hosting night dish. It's quick to prepare but feels special, so you can spend more time enjoying your dinner than standing over the stove. This pasta dish combines sweet crab with a hint of chilli, and courgette to add an extra veggie boost.*

# Crab, Chilli and Courgette Spaghetti

**SERVES 2**
**Under 265kcal,**
**15g protein per serving**

160g (5¾oz) dried spaghetti

Olive oil, for cooking

1 banana shallot,
    finely chopped

2 garlic cloves, minced

1 teaspoon chopped red
    chilli (adjust to taste)

200g (7oz) cherry
    tomatoes, halved

100g (3½oz) white crab meat

1 courgette (zucchini),
    julienned or pared
    into ribbons

Zest and juice of 1 lemon

Salt and pepper

Chopped parsley, to garnish

Grated Parmesan cheese,
    to serve (optional)

Bring a large pan of salted water to the boil. Add the spaghetti and cook according to the packet instructions, until al dente. Drain, reserving about ½ cup of the pasta cooking water.

While the spaghetti is cooking, heat a generous drizzle of olive oil in a large pan over a medium heat. Add the shallot and sauté for 2–3 minutes until softened and translucent. Add the garlic and chilli and cook for another 1–2 minutes until fragrant.

Add the cherry tomatoes and cook for 3–4 minutes until they start to soften and release their juices. Lower the heat to a gentle simmer and mix in the crab meat and courgette. Cook for another 2–3 minutes until the courgette is tender.

Toss the cooked spaghetti into the pan with the crab-tomato mixture. Add the lemon zest and juice and a splash of the reserved pasta water. Stir everything together, allowing the flavours to combine. If the mixture seems too dry, add a little more pasta water until you reach your desired consistency.

Season with salt and pepper to taste and serve, garnished with parsley and topped with a drizzle of olive oil and some grated Parmesan, if desired.

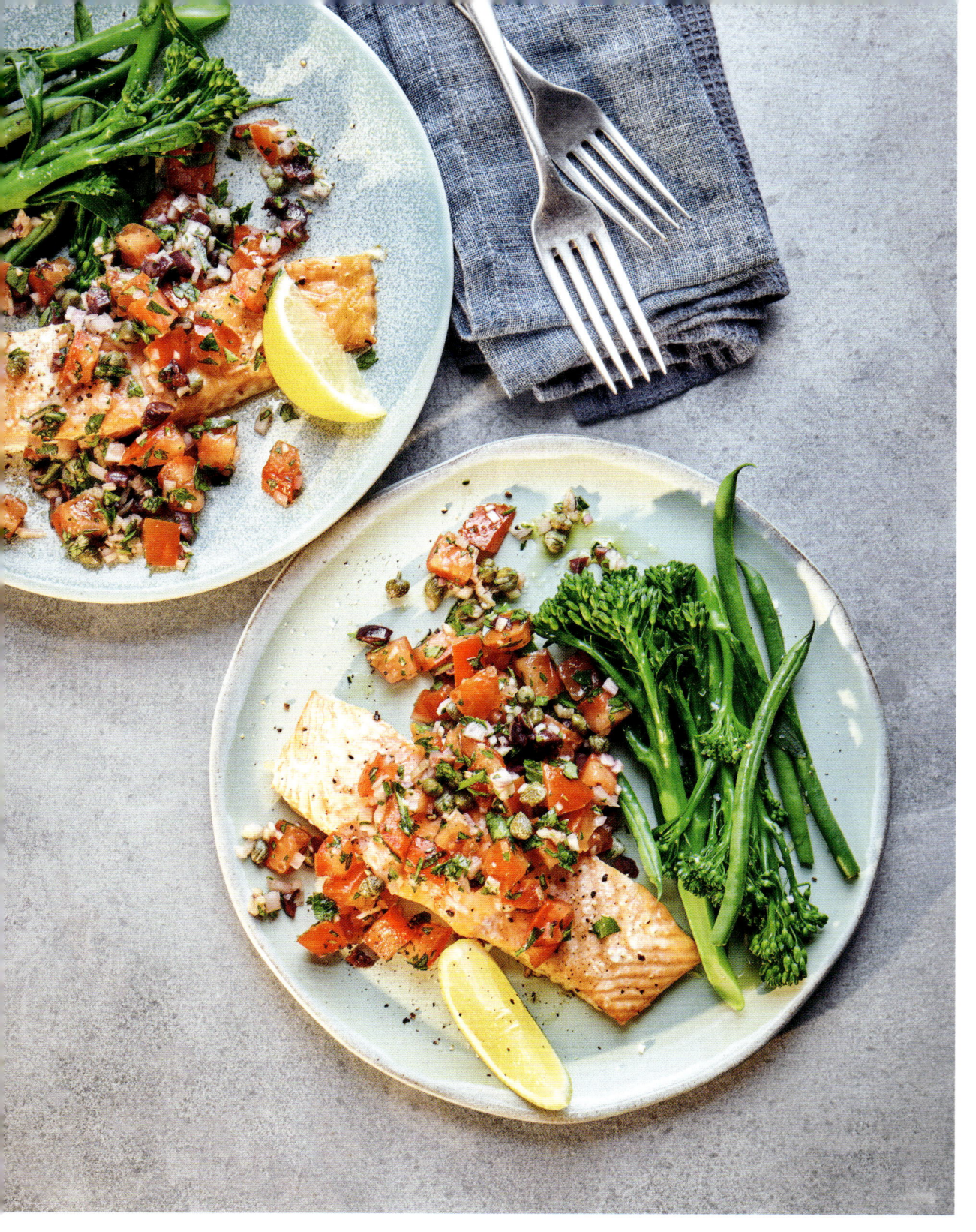

*Sauce vierge is a light, fresh, no-cook sauce packed with healthy fats from olive oil, ripe tomatoes and antioxidant-rich herbs, making it a nutritious addition to any meal. You can easily swap out the salmon for any protein you like, such as chicken, tofu or cod.*

# Baked Salmon with Sauce Vierge

**SERVES 2**
**Under 512kcal,**
**25g protein per serving**

2 skinless salmon fillets
Olive oil, for brushing
Squeeze of lemon juice

**FOR THE SAUCE VIERGE**
2 medium tomatoes, deseeded and roughly chopped into 1 x 1cm (½ inch) pieces
4 tablespoons extra virgin olive oil
Juice of 1 lemon
1 garlic clove, minced
1 small shallot, finely chopped
1 tablespoon capers, toasted in a pan with a little olive oil
1 tablespoon pitted Kalamata olives, chopped
1 tablespoon chopped parsley
1 tablespoon chopped tarragon
1 tablespoon chopped basil
Salt and pepper

Preheat the oven to 220°C/200°C fan (425°F) Gas Mark 7.

Prepare the sauce vierge. In a medium pan, combine the chopped tomatoes, olive oil, lemon juice, garlic, shallot, toasted capers, olives and herbs. Stir to combine and season with salt and pepper to taste. Warm the sauce very gently over low heat for 1–2 minutes just to warm, being careful not to cook. Remove from the heat and let rest for 15 minutes. Season to taste.

Meanwhile, brush the salmon fillets with olive oil and season with salt, pepper and lemon juice. Place on a baking tray lined with nonstick baking paper and bake in the oven for 8–10 minutes, or until the salmon is cooked through and flakes easily with a fork.

To serve, place the baked salmon on plates and spoon 2 tablespoons of the sauce vierge over the top. Serve alongside some sautéed green beans or Tenderstem broccoli.

# Yogurt Harissa Chicken with Smoky Rice

**SERVES 2**
Under 600kcal,
**52g protein per serving**

**FOR THE YOGURT
HARISSA CHICKEN**
2 boneless, skinless
  chicken breasts
3 tablespoons full-fat
  Greek yogurt
1 heaped tablespoon
  harissa paste
2 garlic cloves, minced
Juice of 1 lemon
1 teaspoon salt
½ teaspoon black pepper
1 tablespoon honey

**FOR THE SMOKY RICE**
Olive oil, for cooking
1 red onion, finely sliced
1 red (bell) pepper, cored,
  deseeded and sliced
1 yellow (bell) pepper, cored,
  deseeded and sliced
2 garlic cloves, minced
1 tablespoon harissa paste
1 teaspoon smoked paprika
1 tablespoon tomato
  purée (paste)
100g (3½oz) cherry
  tomatoes, halved
250g (1¾ cups) precooked
  brown rice
Salt and pepper

**TO SERVE**
50g (1¾oz) feta cheese,
  crumbled
Pomegranate seeds
Chopped parsley

Using a rolling pin, slightly hammer out the chicken breasts to an even thickness. In a bowl, mix together the remaining chicken ingredients, add the chicken to coat in the marinade and refrigerate for at least 1 hour, or overnight for best results.

Preheat the oven to 200°C/180°C fan (400°F) Gas Mark 6.

Place the marinated chicken breasts on a baking tray lined with nonstick baking paper and bake for 20–25 minutes until cooked through and the juices run clear. Alternatively, you can grill (broil) the chicken under a medium-high heat for 5–7 minutes on each side until fully cooked. Allow the chicken to rest for 10 minutes before slicing.

While the chicken is cooking, heat a little olive oil in a large pan over a medium heat. Add the red onion and red and yellow peppers. Sauté for 10 minutes until the vegetables are soft and start to caramelise. Add the garlic, harissa paste and smoked paprika and cook for another 2 minutes, stirring frequently.

Stir in the tomato purée and cherry tomatoes and cook for another 3–4 minutes until the tomatoes start to soften. Add the rice with salt and pepper to taste, mixing well to combine with the vegetables and spices. Cook for another 3–5 minutes until the rice is heated through and has absorbed the flavours.

To serve, place a portion of smoky rice on each plate and top with the sliced chicken. Sprinkle the feta, pomegranate seeds and parsley over the chicken and rice.

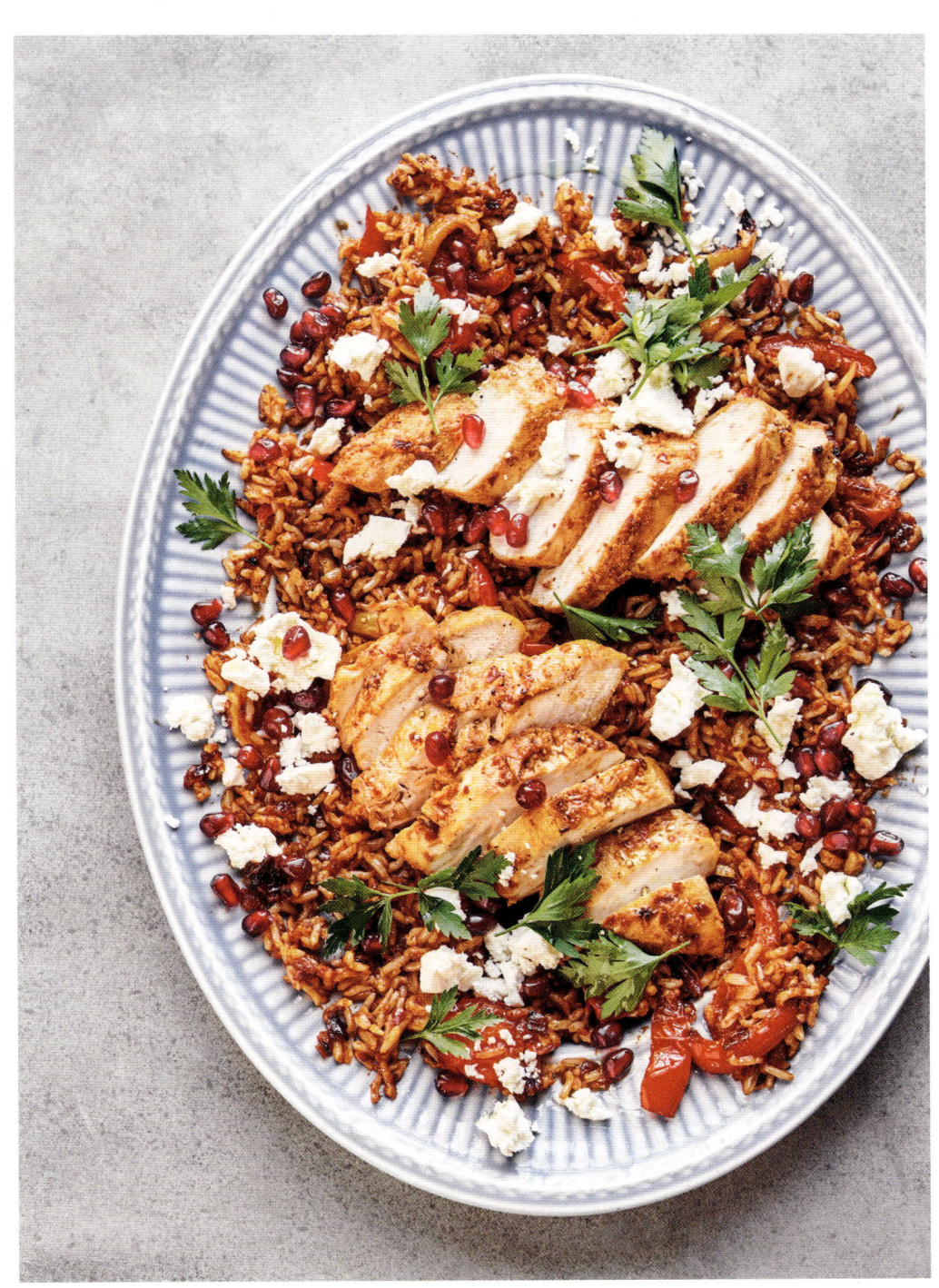

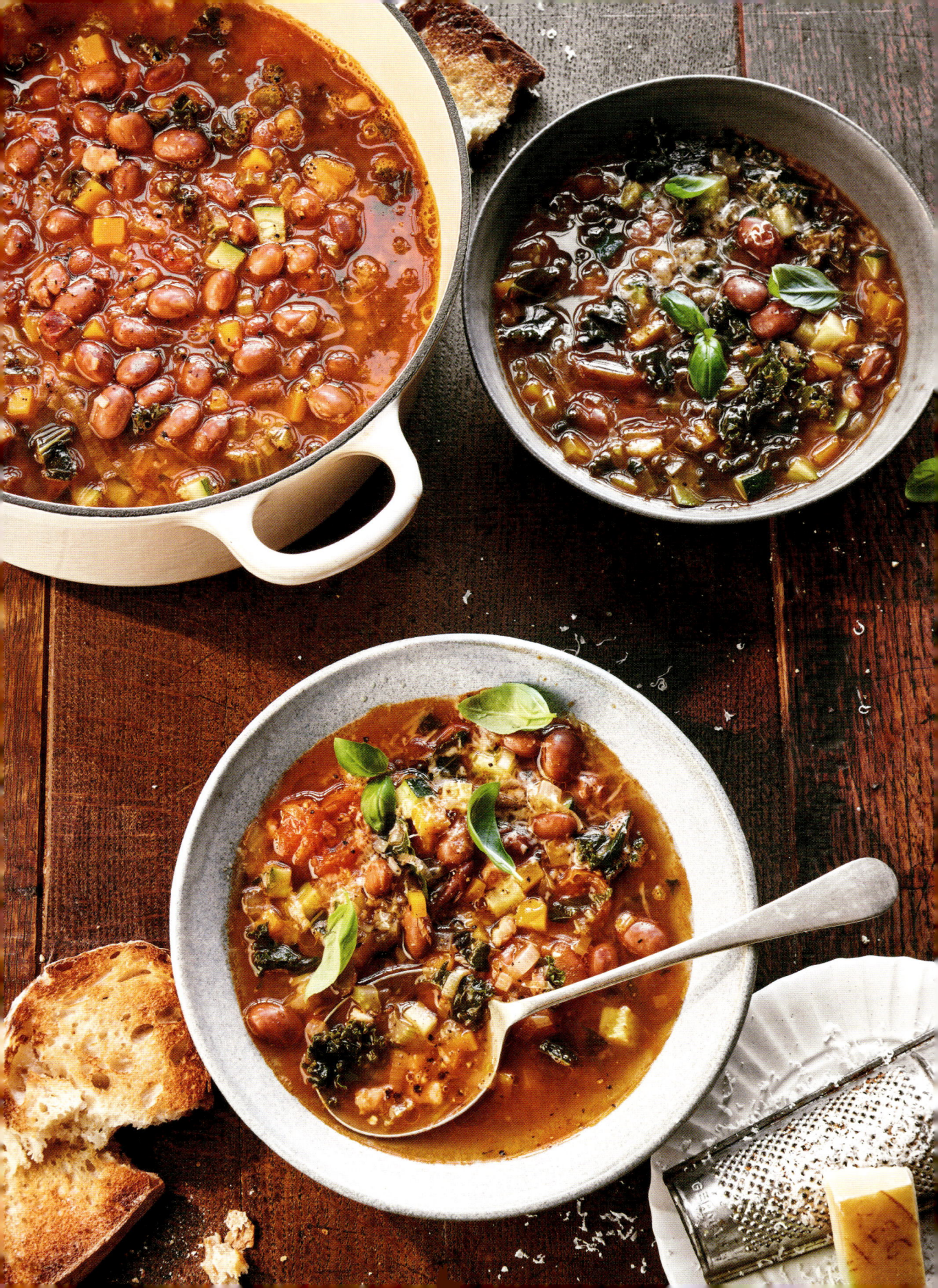

*When you treat and cook vegetables properly, their flavour is next to none. This minestrone is light yet full of layers of different flavours. It can easily be made vegetarian by omitting the pancetta and Parmesan. To boost the protein content you can add some shredded roast chicken.*

# Longevity Minestrone

**SERVES 4**
**Under 390kcal,**
**18g protein per serving**

1 tablespoon olive oil

80g (2¾oz) pancetta or 6 slices of streaky bacon, finely diced

1 red onion, finely diced

3 garlic cloves, minced

2 celery sticks, finely diced

1 leek, trimmed, cleaned and sliced

2 carrots, finely diced

1 courgette (zucchini), cubed

About 1.5 litres (6½ cups) water

2 chicken stock cubes

1 tablespoon tomato purée (paste)

1 tablespoon sun-dried tomato paste

150g (5½oz) cherry tomatoes

30g (1oz) Parmesan cheese, grated, and its rind

2 tablespoons balsamic vinegar

2 x 400g (14oz) cans of beans (borlotti, cannellini, etc.), drained and rinsed

2 handfuls of any finely shredded kale (or other greens)

Good handful of basil leaves, torn

Salt and pepper

Extra virgin olive oil and sourdough bread, to serve

Heat the olive oil in a large pan over a low to medium heat, add the pancetta or bacon, red onion, garlic, celery, leek and carrots and sweat the veg down with a good pinch of salt for around 5 minutes, until softened.

Add the courgette, continuing to sweat down for another 5 minutes, until you see a lovely caramelisation on the bottom of your pan (but make sure the vegetables don't burn). This should be golden, not dark, adding amazing flavour. Once everything has cooked down, pour in enough water to cover all the vegetables by around 2.5cm (1 inch).

Crumble in the stock cubes and add the tomato purée and sun-dried tomato paste, along with a grind of pepper. Bring to the boil then add the cherry tomatoes and Parmesan rind. Place a lid on and let it simmer for 5 minutes over a low heat, adding the balsamic vinegar for acidity. Add the beans and simmer for 20 minutes, then add the shredded kale. Pop the lid back on and cook for 10 minutes until the kale is soft.

Throw in most of the basil then taste, adding pepper, salt, vinegar, etc. if needed.

To serve, spoon the soup into bowls and top with the grated Parmesan, basil and a drizzle of extra virgin olive oil. Serve with a slab of toasted sourdough.

# Get Ahead Marinades

Let's be honest – sometimes we just need something quick and tasty to throw into a meal without overthinking. That's where these marinades come in. They're my go-to for prepping proteins ahead of time, so they're ready to cook whenever you are. Whether you're grilling chicken, roasting fish or pan-frying tofu, these marinades are packed with flavour and make life so much easier.

The best part? They freeze beautifully! I like to portion the marinated protein into freezer bags (flat, so they defrost faster). You can also keep them in the refrigerator if you're planning to use them sooner – just make sure you use them within 2–3 days to keep everything fresh. Try these and your future self will thank you when dinner is sorted in no time. No boring meals here – just quick, tasty dinners that feel way fancier than the effort you put in.

## HOW TO MAKE THEM WORK FOR YOU

**Freeze in Portions:** I always portion my marinated protein into single-use bags or containers; they can be frozen for up to 3 months. Flatten the bags – they defrost more quickly that way.

**Cook Straight from Frozen:** Most of the marinated proteins work great straight from the freezer. Just toss them in the oven, onto a grill (broiler) or into a pan.

**Beyond Proteins:** Use these marinades as a dressing for vegetables or as a sauce base. The coconut and lemongrass marinade is amazing over rice or noodles.

# Jalapeño, Honey and Lime Marinade

1 fresh jalapeño, diced

Juice of 1 lime

Large handful of coriander (cilantro) leaves

1 garlic clove, peeled

1 teaspoon honey

2 spring onions (scallions), trimmed

Salt, to taste

*Zingy, fresh and with just the right amount of spice, this marinade is perfect for prawns, chicken or tofu.*

Blend all the ingredients together in a blender or food processor until smooth. Pour over the protein, mix to coat and marinate for at least 30 minutes – or store in the refrigerator for up to 2 days.

# Yogurt Harissa Marinade

2 heaped tablespoons Greek yogurt

1 heaped teaspoon harissa paste

1 garlic clove, peeled

Juice of 1 lemon

½ red onion, roughly chopped

1 teaspoon smoked honey

½ teaspoon chilli powder

Salt, to taste

*Creamy, smoky and with a kick of heat, this marinade is incredible for chicken thighs or lamb.*

Blend all the ingredients together in a blender or food processor until smooth. Pour over the protein, mix to coat and marinate for at least an hour – or store in the refrigerator for up to 2 days.

# Coconut and Lemongrass Marinade

150ml (⅔ cup) coconut milk

1 stick lemongrass, roughly chopped

1 garlic clove, peeled

2 spring onions (scallions), trimmed

1 tablespoon Thai red curry paste

1 tablespoon soy sauce

1 teaspoon ginger paste

*Silky, fragrant and with those classic Thai-inspired flavours, this marinade is perfect for chicken, fish or prawns.*

Blend all the ingredients together in a blender or food processor until smooth. Pour over the protein, mix to coat and marinate for at least an hour – or store in the refrigerator for up to 3 days.

*Aubergine can be a love-it-or-hate-it food. Here, I slice and bake it quickly as a healthier alternative to frying. Once softened, the slices are filled with a zesty, punchy spinach and ricotta mixture, rolled, then covered with a simple tomato sauce and a layer of cheese. This is comfort food without compromising on your health.*

# Aubergine Cannelloni with Garlic and Herb Crumb

**SERVES 2**

**Under 480kcal,**
**25g protein per serving**

1 aubergine (eggplant)
   – shorter and fatter
   works better here

Olive oil, for brushing
   and cooking

200g (7oz) baby spinach leaves

250g (1 cup) ricotta cheese

40g (1½oz) Parmesan
   cheese, grated

Zest of 1 lemon

Salt and pepper

**FOR THE TOMATO SAUCE**

1 banana shallot,
   finely chopped

1 red (bell) pepper,
   cored, deseeded and
   finely chopped

2 garlic cloves, minced

400g (14oz) can of
   chopped tomatoes

1 tablespoon sun-dried
   tomato paste

Handful of basil leaves, torn

**FOR THE GARLIC AND**
**HERB CRUMB**

2 slices of leftover sourdough
   (about 80g/2¾oz)

1 garlic clove, minced

2 teaspoons extra
   virgin olive oil

1 tablespoon each of basil
   and parsley leaves

Preheat the oven to 220°C/200°C fan (425°F) Gas Mark 7.

Slice the aubergine lengthways into 5mm (¼ inch) slices – not too thick but not too thin. Brush both sides with a little olive oil, lay flat on a baking tray and bake in the oven for 15 minutes, turning once until just softened but still firm enough to hold the filling.

Rinse the spinach then add to a pan and wilt over a medium heat. Squeeze all the moisture out, season with a little salt and pepper, then roughly chop.

Mix the spinach into the ricotta, aiming for a 50:50 ratio. Season with the Parmesan, lemon zest and plenty of pepper. Taste and adjust the seasoning as needed.

To make the simple tomato sauce, heat a little olive oil in a pan over a low to medium heat, add the shallot and red pepper and sweat them down for a few minutes with a little salt. Add the garlic and cook until softened, then add the chopped tomatoes, sun-dried tomato paste and a splash of water. Simmer until thickened, then season with pepper and add the basil.

For the garlic and herb crumb, pulse the ingredients together in a food processor to create breadcrumbs.

Lay an aubergine slice flat, add a generous spoonful of the ricotta mixture into the centre and roll up to form a tube. Add a thin layer of tomato sauce to the bottom of a baking dish. Lay the aubergine rolls on top, sealed side down, side by side. Continue until all the slices are used up.

Top the rolls with the remaining tomato sauce and cover with the breadcrumb mix. Bake for 20–25 minutes until golden and bubbling. I like to serve this with a nice side salad.

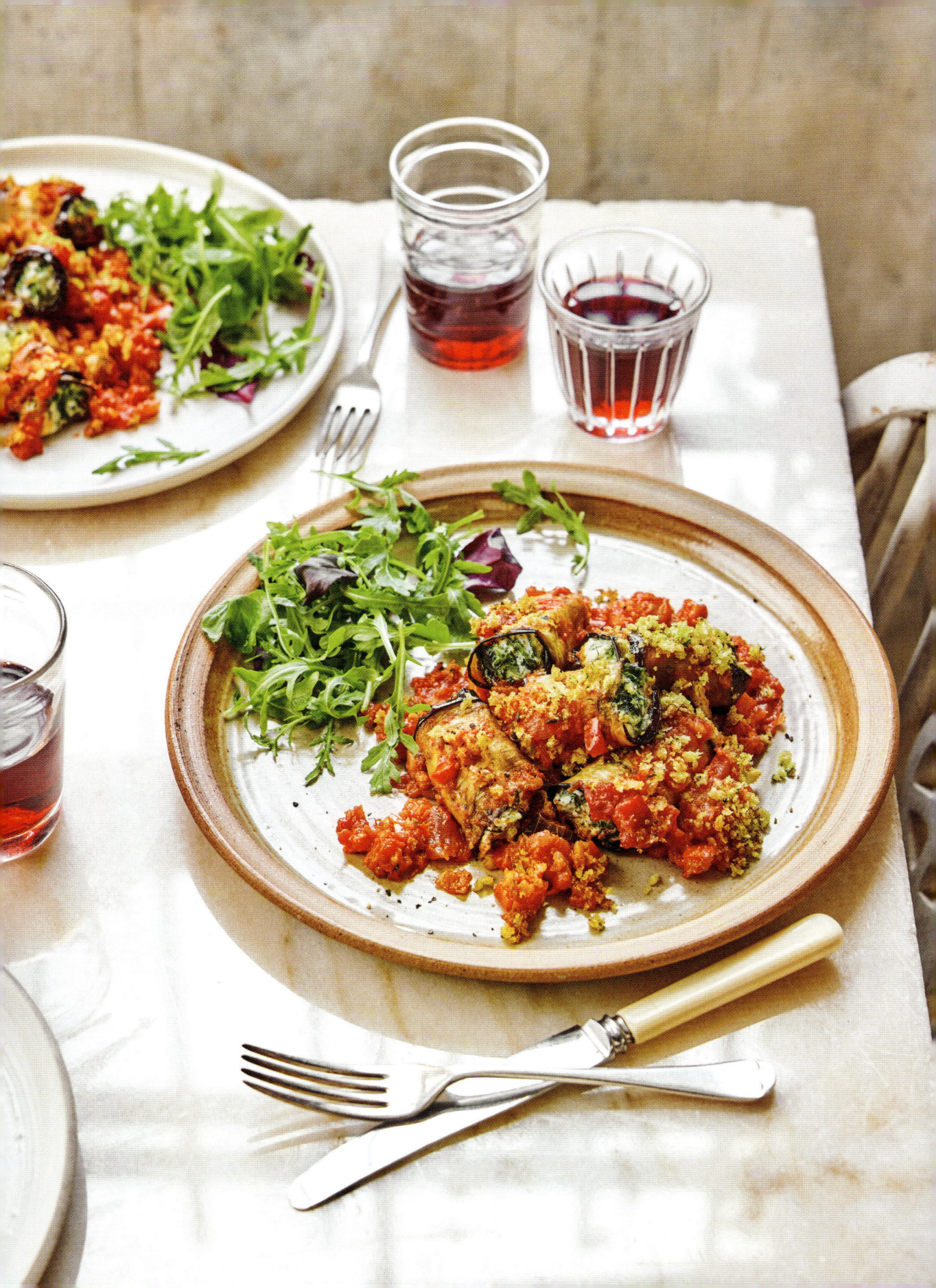

*This is one of my favourite quick and easy meals to make when I don't want to spend a long time in the kitchen. Perfect for meal prep, but just keep the feta separate and heat up at work. You can easily swap the chicken for any protein you like.*

# Loaded Harissa Chicken Potatoes with Herby Feta

**SERVES 1**
**Under 540kcal,**
**42g protein per serving**

1 small sweet potato (about 180g/6½oz)

Olive oil, for rubbing and cooking

½ red onion, sliced

1 teaspoon harissa paste

½ red (bell) pepper, deseeded and sliced

Handful of cherry tomatoes, halved

120g (4oz) cooked chicken breast, shredded (or any protein you like)

1 tablespoon tomato purée (paste)

1 tablespoon balsamic vinegar

Salt and pepper

**FOR THE HERBY FETA**

Handful of parsley leaves, finely chopped

Zest of ½ lemon

30g (1oz) feta cheese

Preheat the oven to 200°C/180°C fan (400°F) Gas Mark 6.

Rub the sweet potato with olive oil and salt and pierce it a few times with a fork to allow steam to escape. Microwave on high for 5 minutes to soften it, then transfer to the oven and bake for 10 minutes until the skin is crispy and the potato is tender inside.

While the sweet potato is cooking, heat a drizzle of olive oil in a pan over a medium heat. Add the red onion and sauté with a pinch of salt until it softens, about 3 minutes. Add the harissa paste and cook for another minute until fragrant.

Add the red pepper and cherry tomatoes to the pan. Sauté for 5 minutes until they start to soften. Add the shredded chicken and tomato purée, stirring to combine. Add a splash of water, along with the balsamic vinegar, to create a sauce. Continue to cook for another 5–7 minutes until the mixture is thick and well combined. Season with salt and pepper to taste.

While the chicken mixture is simmering, prepare the herby feta. Place the parsley and lemon zest in a small bowl and crumble in the feta. Mix everything until it is well combined.

Cut open the cooked sweet potato and fluff the inside with a fork. Top with the harissa chicken mixture. Scatter the herby feta over the top and serve immediately.

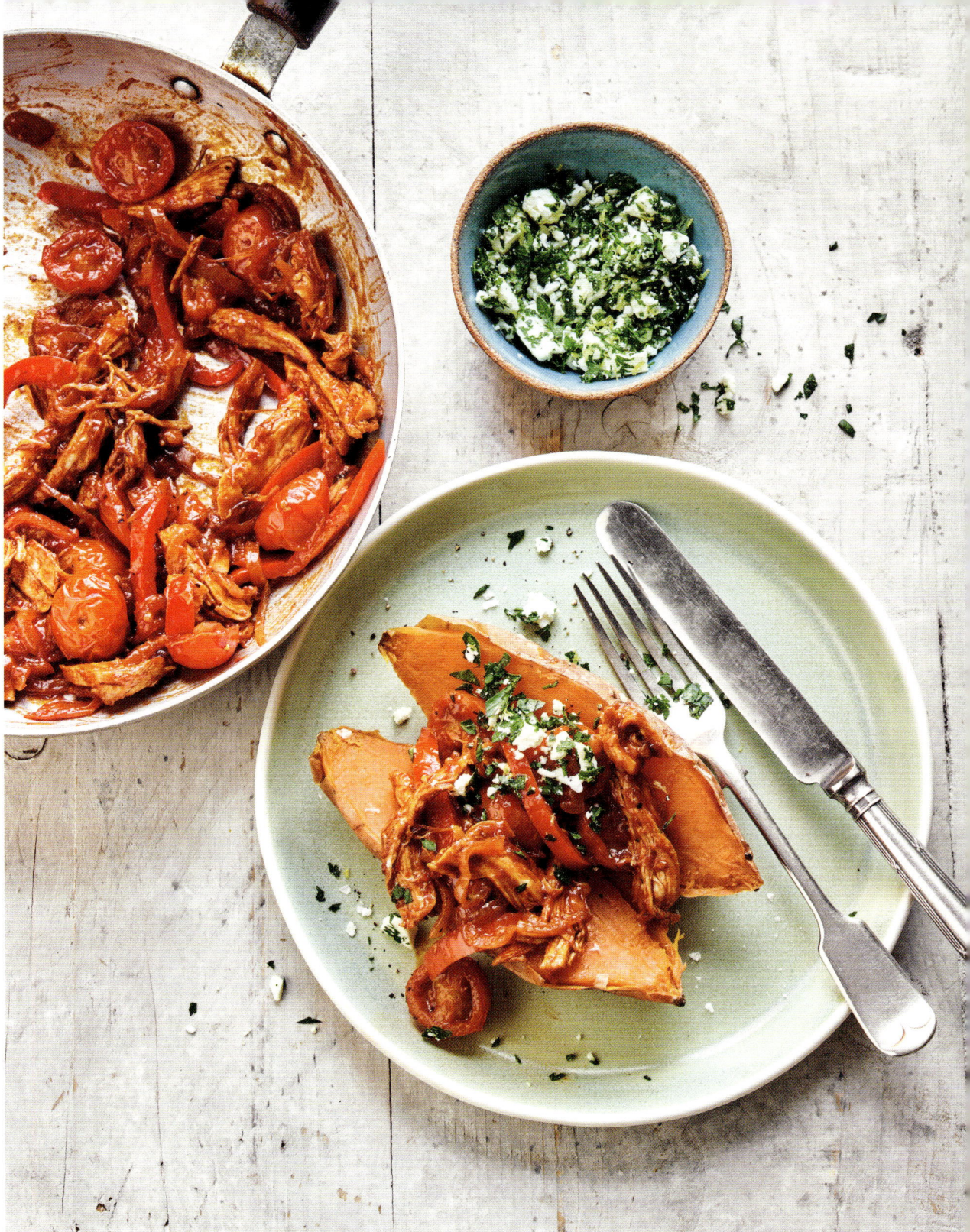

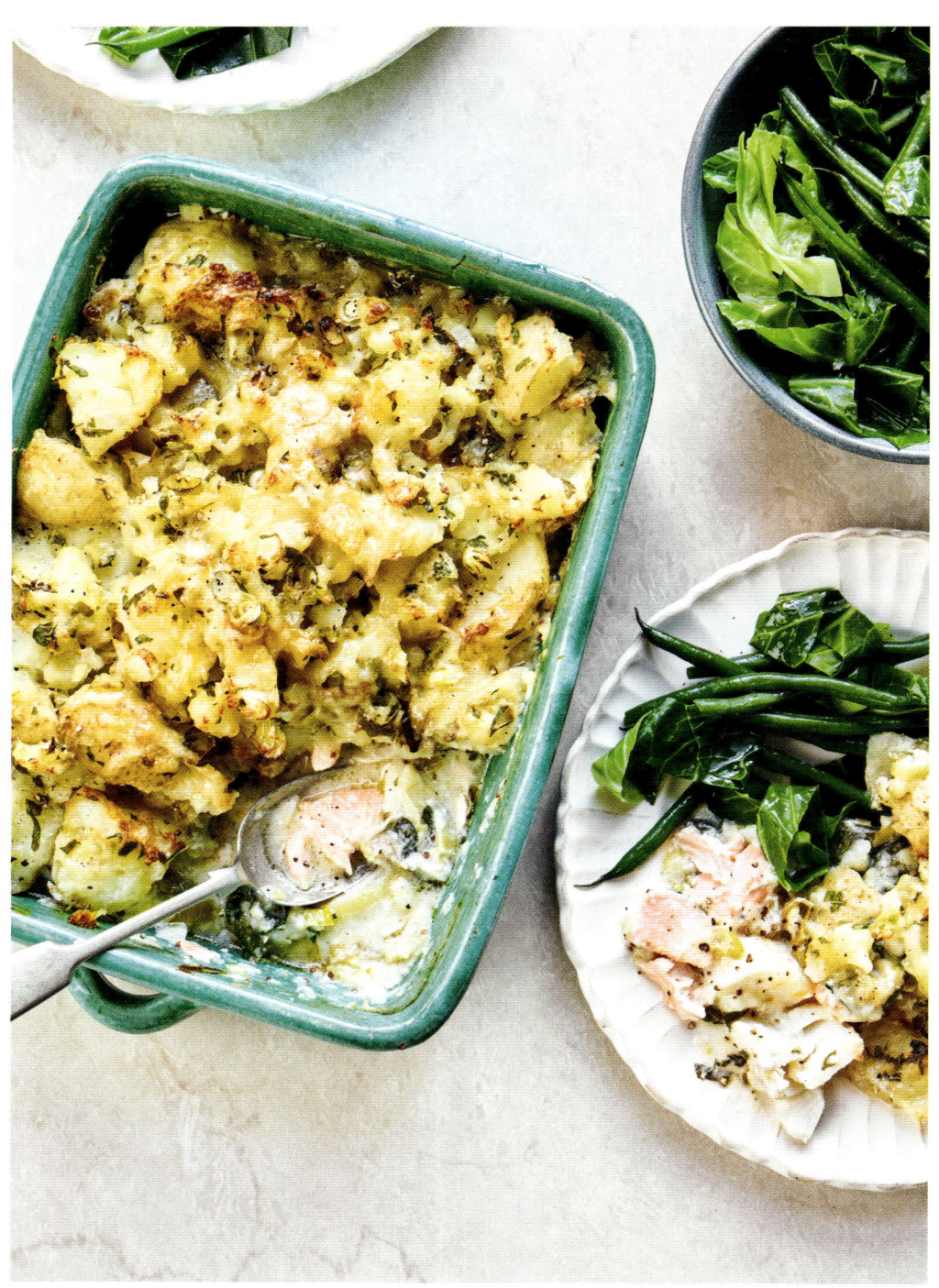

*A comforting and nutritious fish pie mix but with a crispy potato top that's much better than mash, in my opinion. Crushed just-boiled potatoes with olive oil, cheese, lots of parsley and spring onion topped on to a creamy leek and fish pie mix and baked until golden and gorgeous. Just so good.*

# Crispy Potato Fish Pie Bake

**SERVES 4**
**Under 380kcal,**
**30g protein per serving**

Olive oil, for cooking

1 leek, trimmed, cleaned and finely sliced

2 garlic cloves, minced

2 tablespoons plain (all-purpose) flour

500ml (generous 2 cups) milk (any kind)

1 chicken stock cube

1 tablespoon wholegrain mustard

Handful of baby spinach leaves

350–400g (12–14oz) fish pie mix (a combination of salmon, cod and smoked haddock)

Salt and pepper

Steamed green beans, to serve

**FOR THE CRISPY POTATO TOPPING**

500g (1lb 2oz) skin-on baby potatoes, halved or quartered

Sprig of rosemary

2 or 3 garlic cloves, smashed

70g (2½oz) smoked Cheddar cheese, grated

1 tablespoon olive oil

2 spring onions (scallions), chopped

Large handful of parsley leaves, chopped

Preheat the oven to 200°C/180°C fan (400°F) Gas Mark 6.

Add the baby potatoes to a large pan and fill with water to cover. Season with salt, add the rosemary and garlic cloves, bring to a simmer and cook until the potatoes are tender and a knife goes through them easily. Drain and return to the pan, or transfer to a bowl. Discard the garlic and rosemary.

As the potatoes cook, heat another pan over a medium heat. Add a drizzle of olive oil and sweat the leek and garlic with a pinch each of salt and pepper until soft, about 5–7 minutes.

Sprinkle in the flour, mix, and slowly whisk in the milk until fully combined. Bring the mixture to a simmer to thicken, then crumble in the stock cube and add the mustard. Simmer for a few minutes, then add the spinach and mix until wilted. Take off the heat.

Fold the fish into the sauce and pour the mixture into a suitable baking dish (or bake in the same pan if it is ovenproof).

Add 40g (1½oz) of the grated Cheddar to the potatoes, with the olive oil, spring onions, parsley and salt and pepper to taste. Using a spoon, roughly mash the potatoes, leaving nice chunky pieces.

Top the fish mixture with the potato, spreading it evenly. Sprinkle the remaining grated Cheddar over the top and bake in the oven for 20–25 minutes until the top is golden brown and crispy. Serve with steamed green beans.

*I love a good burger, and these ones with lamb and feta are a perfect flavourful yet balanced dinner option. They are quick to make, prepable and freezer-friendly. The addition of grated courgettes keeps them juicy and light. Served with a cucumber slaw and a dollop of garlic yogurt, these will become a family favourite. I've paired them with garlic lemon potato wedges for a complete meal.*

# Lamb and Feta Burgers with Cucumber Slaw and Garlic Yogurt

**SERVES 4**
**Under 590kcal,**
**44g protein per serving**

Olive oil, for cooking

500g (1lb 2oz) lean minced (ground) lamb

1 small courgette (zucchini), grated and excess water squeezed out

80g (2¾oz) feta cheese

1 teaspoon garlic granules

1 teaspoon onion granules

Zest of 1 lemon

Pinch of dried rosemary

4 burger rolls

Salt and pepper

**FOR THE GARLIC LEMON POTATO WEDGES**

500g (1lb 2oz) skin-on potatoes, cut into wedges

½ teaspoon garlic granules

Zest and juice of 1 lemon

1 teaspoon dried rosemary

**FOR THE CUCUMBER LEMON MINT SLAW**

½ cucumber, pared into ribbons

Zest and juice of ½ lemon

1 tablespoon mint, chopped

**FOR THE GARLIC YOGURT**

100g (scant ½ cup) thick Greek yogurt (0% or full fat)

¼ teaspoon garlic granules

1 tablespoon mint, chopped

Preheat the oven to 200°C/180°C fan (400°F) Gas Mark 6.

In a large bowl, toss the potato wedges with 1 tablespoon of olive oil, the garlic granules, lemon zest and juice, dried rosemary and some salt and pepper. Spread the wedges in a single layer on a baking tray and roast in the oven for 25–30 minutes, turning halfway through, until golden brown and crispy.

Meanwhile, in a bowl, combine the minced lamb, courgette, garlic granules, onion granules, lemon zest, dried rosemary, 1 teaspoon of salt and a grind of pepper. Crumble in the feta. Gently fold the mixture together until well combined. Shape into 4 equal-sized patties.

Mix the cucumber ribbons in a small bowl with the lemon zest and juice and mint. Season with salt and pepper to taste and set aside.

In another small bowl, combine the yogurt with the garlic granules, mint and a pinch each of salt and pepper. Mix well and set aside.

Heat a little olive oil in a frying pan over a medium heat. Fry the lamb burgers until golden brown and cooked through, about 4–5 minutes on each side. While the burgers cook, toast the burger buns in the oven or grill (broiler).

Spread some garlic yogurt on the bottom half of each toasted bun and add a lamb burger. Top with a generous spoonful of cucumber slaw. Add a little extra garlic yogurt to the top bun and place it on top. Serve the lamb and feta burgers with the potato wedges on the side.

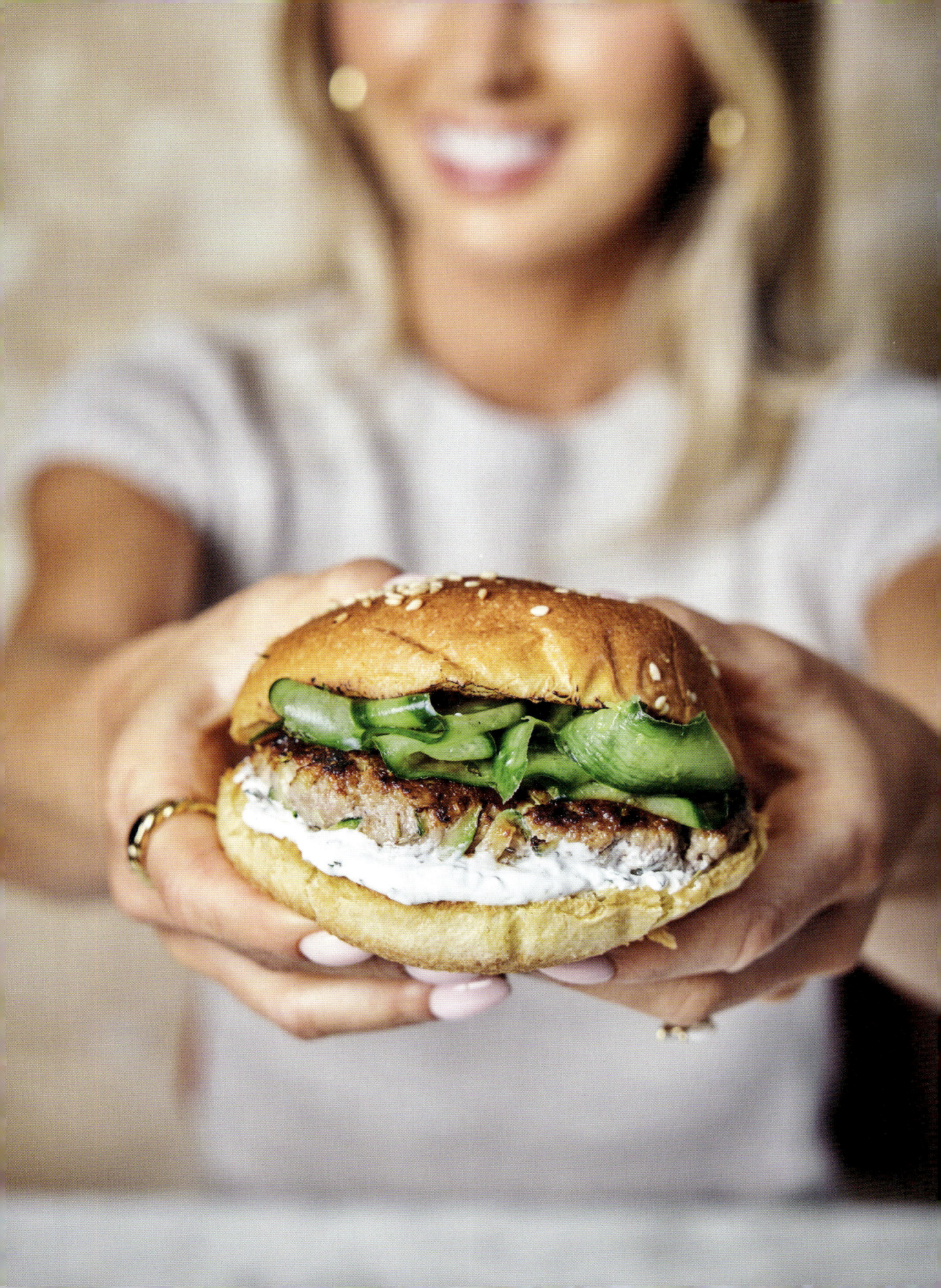

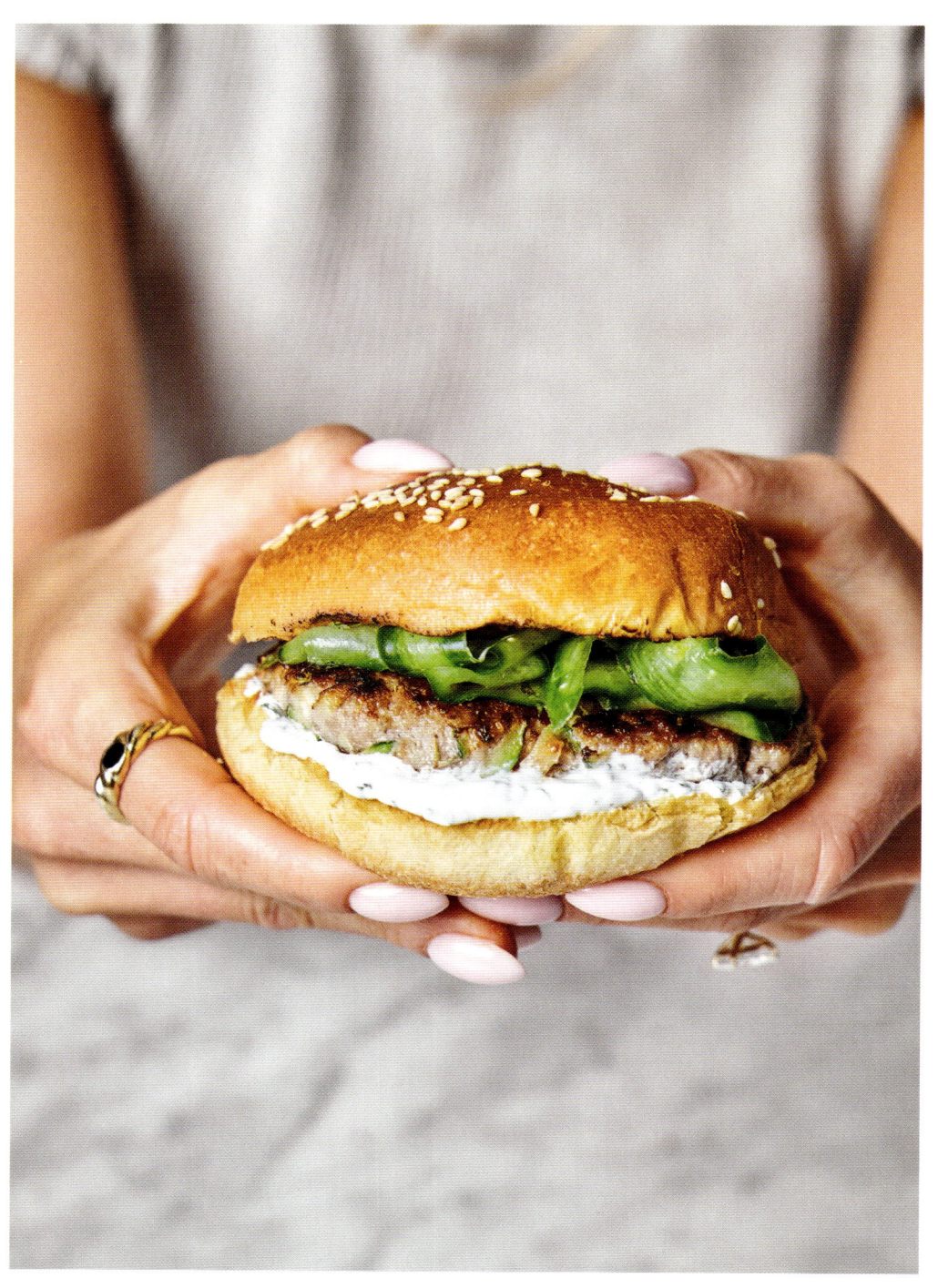

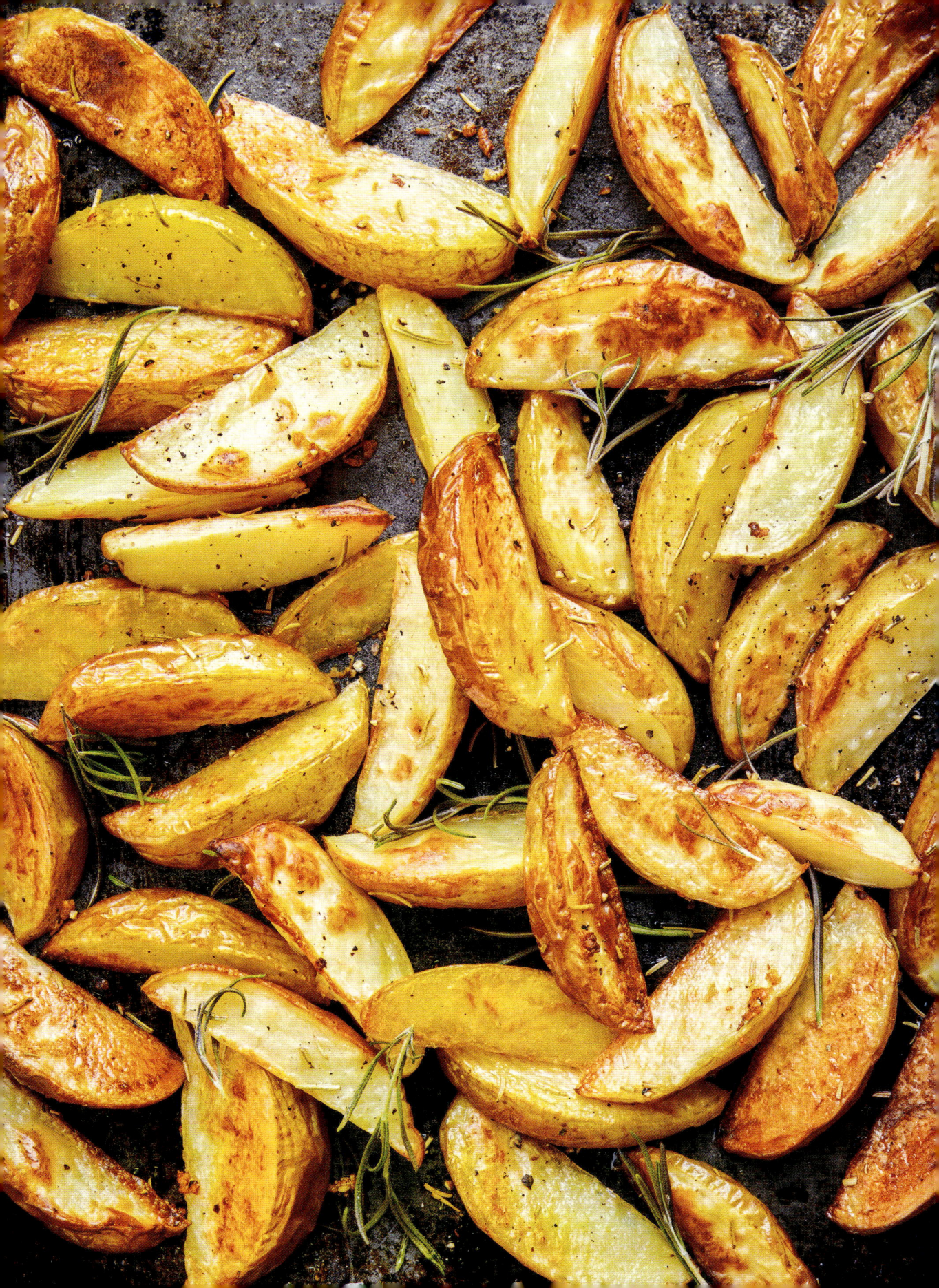

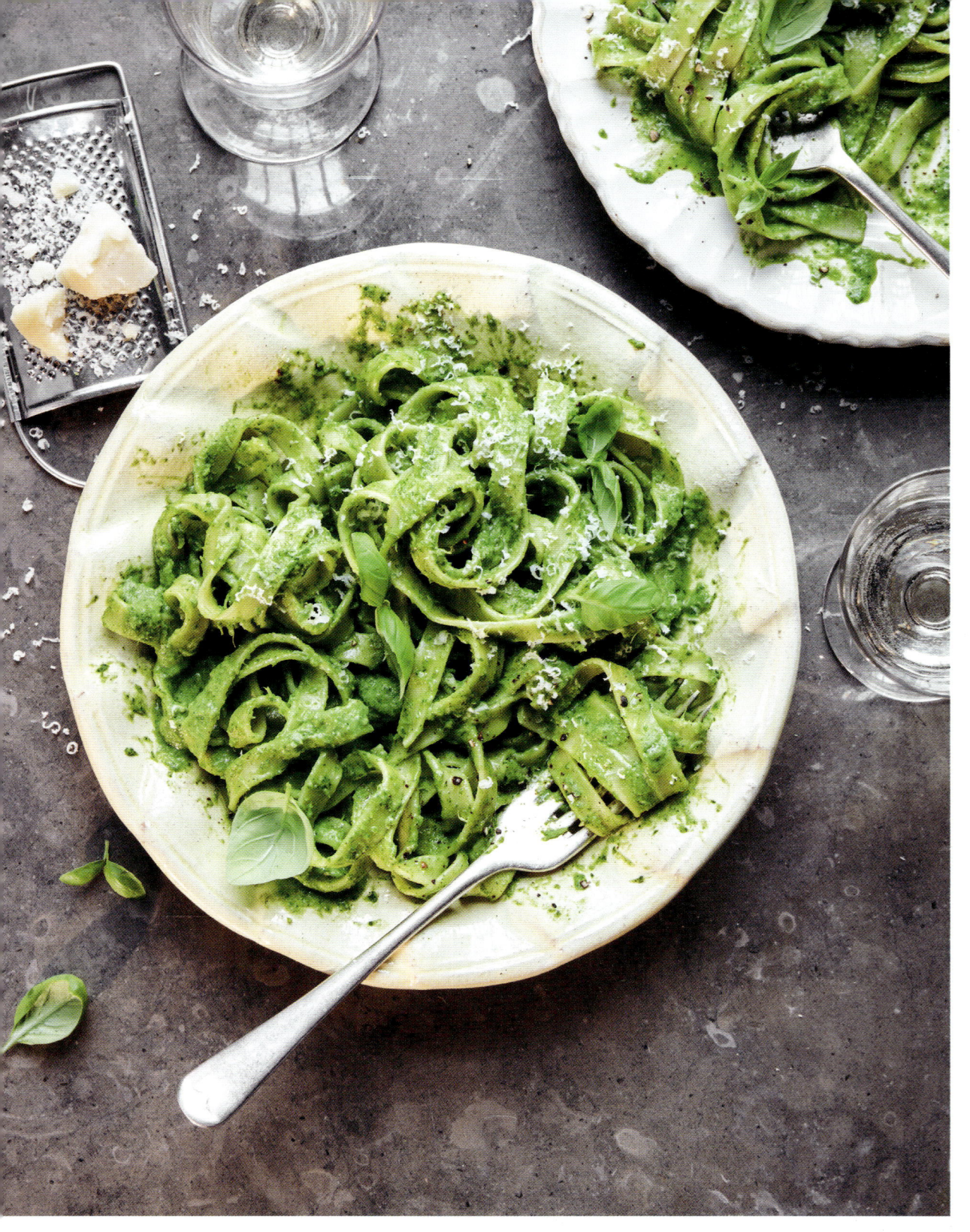

*This is one of those recipes that packs in all the goodness in my favourite form – a big bowl of pasta. It has the silkiest vibrant green sauce with lots of fresh basil, Parmesan, kale, protein-packed peas and, of course, lots of garlic. Serve with any protein of choice.*

# Simple Super Greens Pasta

**SERVES 2**
**Under 500kcal,**
**22g protein per serving**

150g (5½oz) dried pasta
Olive oil, for cooking
1 shallot, diced
2 garlic cloves, minced
1 leek, trimmed, cleaned and finely sliced
½ teaspoon chopped rosemary leaves
3 large handfuls of kale
120g (1 cup) frozen peas
1 chicken stock cube, crumbled
75ml (5 tablespoons) semi-skimmed milk
40g (1½oz) Parmesan cheese, grated
20g (¾oz) basil leaves
Salt and pepper

Cook the pasta in a pan of salted boiling water until al dente, according to the packet instructions, then drain, reserving a cup of pasta cooking water.

Meanwhile, add a little olive oil to a pan over a low to medium heat and sweat the shallot, garlic, leek and rosemary, with a pinch of salt, until translucent. Add in the kale and frozen peas, mix well, and cover with a lid to steam slightly for 5 minutes, or until the kale is cooked.

Tip the mixture into a powerful blender and add the stock cube, milk, Parmesan, basil and a pinch of pepper. Blend until smooth and vibrant, adding a little more milk if it needs loosening further.

Mix the sauce into the drained pasta. If the sauce becomes too thick, add a little of the reserved pasta water to achieve the desired consistency.

Serve immediately, optionally topped with your protein of choice.

*This Mexican white bean chilli is one of my new favourite meals to eat when I want to sit down with a big bowl of something comforting. It's smoky, creamy, packed full of nutrition and everything you want to eat. Simply sauté it all in a big pot until bubbling and gorgeous, add in a dollop of sour cream and serve with coriander, avocado, feta and lots of lime.*

# Smoky Mexican White Bean Chilli

**SERVES 2**
**Under 366kcal,**
**35g protein per serving**

Olive oil, for cooking

1 onion, finely diced

1 fresh jalapeño pepper, diced (use 2 if you like more heat)

2 garlic cloves, minced

1 teaspoon smoked paprika

1 teaspoon dried oregano

1 green (bell) pepper, cored, deseeded and finely diced

400g (14oz) can of cannellini beans, drained and rinsed

1 chicken stock cube

100g (¾ cup) frozen sweetcorn

200g (7oz) cooked chicken breast, shredded

1 tablespoon cornflour (cornstarch) mixed with 2 tablespoons water, to make a slurry

2 tablespoons sour cream

Juice of ½ lime, plus extra (optional) to serve

Salt and pepper

**TO SERVE (OPTIONAL)**

Chopped coriander (cilantro) leaves

Crumbled feta cheese

Sliced avocado

Heat a little olive oil in a deep pan over a medium heat, then sweat the onion with a pinch of salt for a few minutes, until softened. Add the jalapeño and garlic and sauté for 3 more minutes.

Add the smoked paprika, dried oregano and green pepper. Stir to combine, then tip in the cannellini beans, crumble in the stock cube and cover with just enough water to submerge everything. Add the frozen sweetcorn and shredded chicken and bring to a gentle simmer.

Add the cornflour slurry to the simmering mixture and stir, allowing it to gently thicken for 4–5 minutes.

Stir in the sour cream and lime juice, then season with more salt and pepper to taste.

Serve in bowls. If desired, top with coriander, extra lime, crumbled feta and sliced avocado.

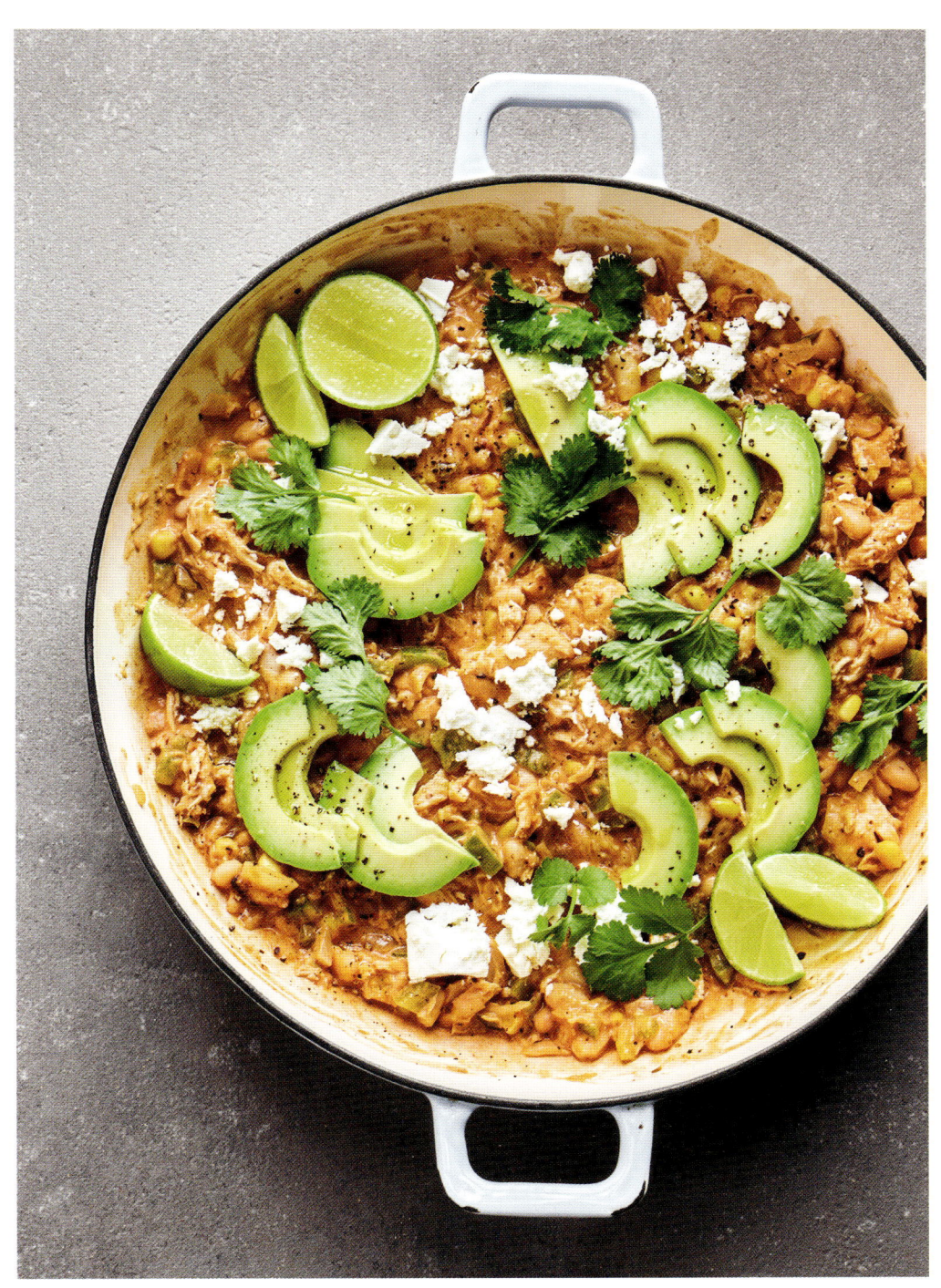

*Proper comfort food, these meatballs are inspired by one of my favourite childhood meals of pork and apple sausages with mashed potatoes. This is my version – full of balance but still hearty and satisfying, perfect for meal prep or a cosy family dinner.*

# Pork and Caramelised Apple Meatballs

**SERVES 4**
**Under 480kcal,**
**40g protein per serving**

Olive oil, for cooking

2 small dessert apples, cored and cut into small cubes

1 onion, finely diced

500g (1lb 2oz) lean minced (ground) pork

50g (1 cup) fresh breadcrumbs

1 medium free-range egg

1 teaspoon garlic granules

1 teaspoon honey

1 teaspoon wholegrain mustard

Salt and pepper

Lemon zest and chopped parsley, to finish

**FOR THE SAUCE**

1 leek, trimmed and sliced

2 garlic cloves, minced

250g (9oz) chestnut mushrooms, sliced

2 sprigs of thyme

2 tablespoons plain (all-purpose) flour

500ml (generous 2 cups) chicken stock

1 teaspoon wholegrain mustard

1 heaped tablespoon half-fat crème fraîche

**FOR THE MASHED POTATOES**

500g (1lb 2oz) potatoes, peeled and cut into chunks

1 tablespoon extra virgin olive oil or butter

75ml (5 tablespoons) milk

**FOR THE GARLIC GREENS**

2 garlic cloves, minced

200g (7oz) greens, such as kale or cavolo nero, shredded

Heat a little olive oil in a pan over a medium heat and sweat the apples and onion until they start to caramelise but still hold their shape, about 7–10 minutes. Tip into a large bowl.

Add the minced pork, breadcrumbs, egg, garlic granules, honey and mustard. Mix well, then shape into golf-ball-sized meatballs. Add a little more oil to the same pan and brown the meatballs on all sides. Remove and set aside.

For the sauce, add the leek, garlic, mushrooms and thyme, and cook for 5 minutes until the vegetables are softened. Sprinkle the flour over the vegetables and stir well to combine.

Gradually whisk in the stock, ensuring there are no lumps. Bring the mixture to a gentle simmer and let it thicken for ten minutes, then add the mustard and crème fraîche. Season with salt and pepper to taste.

Add the meatballs back to the pan and simmer gently for another 10 minutes or until cooked through. Finish with a sprinkle of lemon zest and chopped parsley for freshness.

For the mashed potatoes, place the potato chunks in a large pan and cover with cold water. Add a pinch of salt, bring to the boil and cook until tender, about 15 minutes. Drain, return the potatoes to the pan, add the oil or butter and the milk, and mash until smooth. Season with salt and pepper to taste.

For the greens, heat 1 tablespoon of olive oil in a pan over a medium heat. Add the garlic and sauté for about 1 minute until fragrant. Add the greens and toss to coat, then add a splash of water and place a lid on top. Cook for 4–5 minutes until the greens are tender. Season with salt and pepper to taste.

Serve the meatballs with the mashed potatoes and garlic greens.

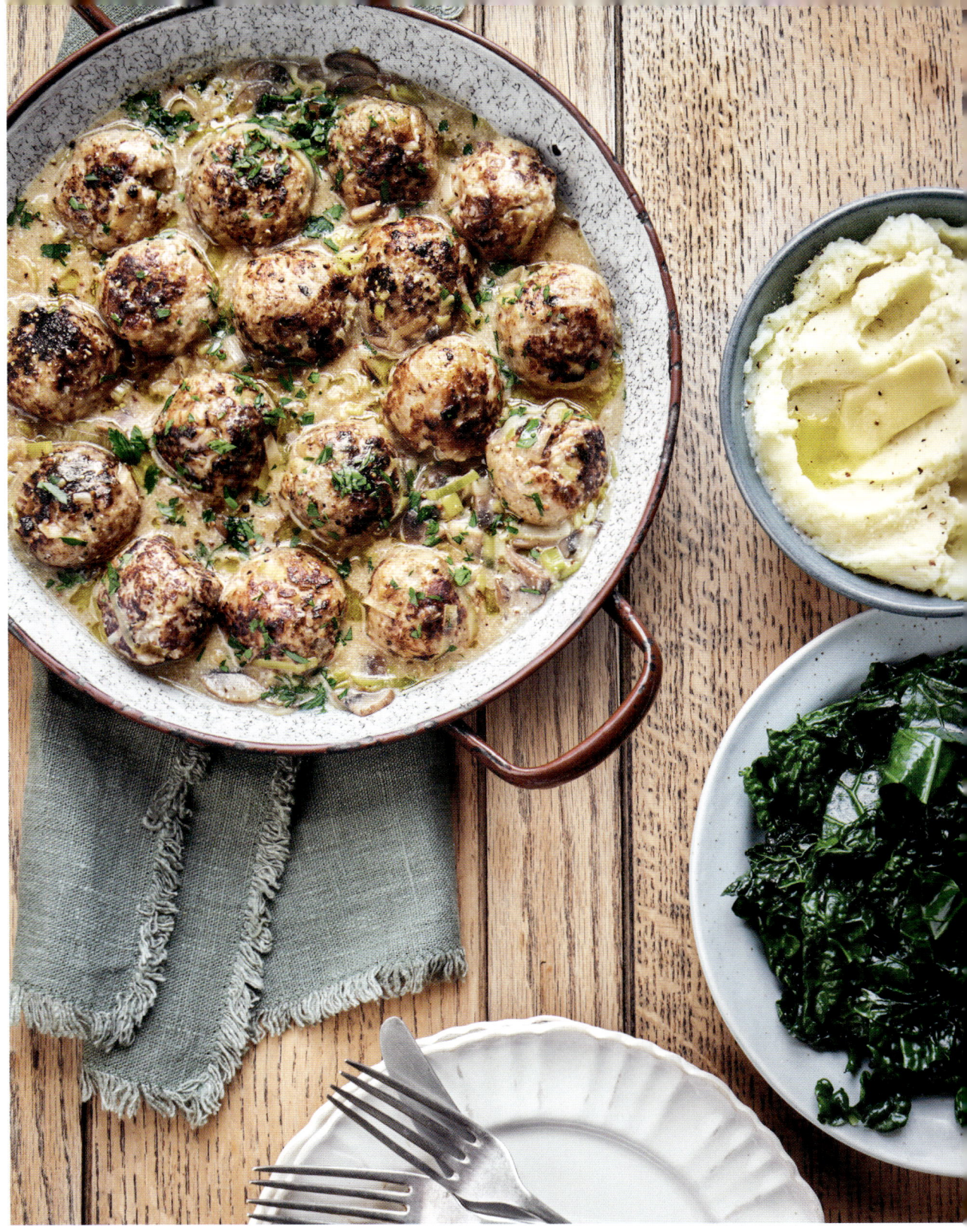

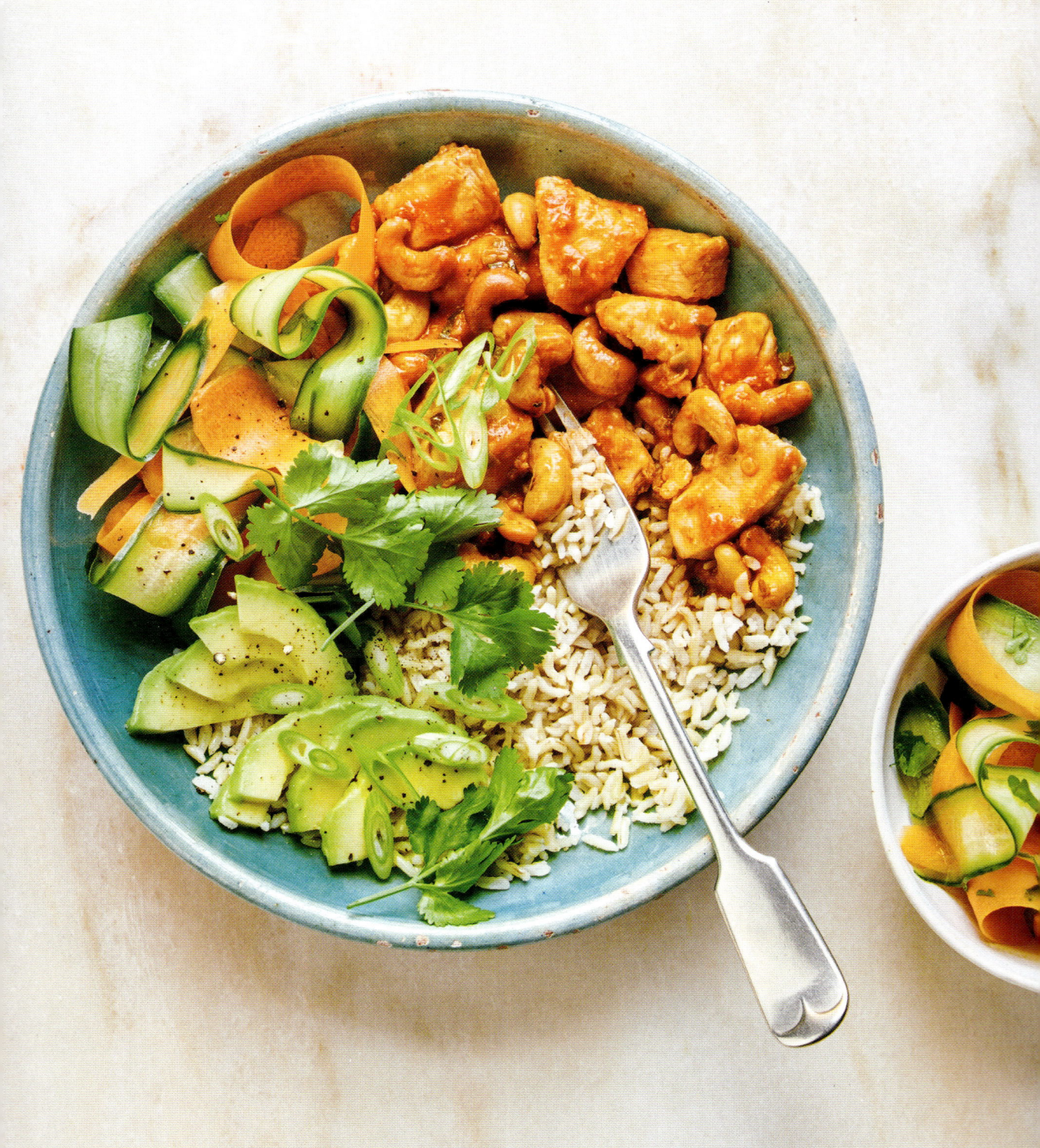

*If you love sweet and sour chicken, you will adore my orange and cashew chicken. Sticky, salty but much lower in sugar, the sauce is sweetened with fresh orange juice only. It's really quick to make, ready in under 15 minutes. Perfect for meal prep and makes fantastic lunch leftovers.*

# Sticky Orange and Cashew Chicken Bowls

**SERVES 2**
**Under 645kcal,**
**54g protein per serving**

300g (10½oz) boneless, skinless chicken breast, diced

1 tablespoon cornflour (cornstarch)

½ cucumber, pared into ribbons

2 carrots, pared into ribbons

1 teaspoon rice vinegar

Small handful of coriander (cilantro) leaves, roughly chopped

250g (2 cups) precooked rice or 120g (¾ cup) uncooked

1 teaspoon neutral oil

2 spring onions (scallions), diced

Small handful of cashew nuts

½ medium ripe avocado, peeled, pitted and sliced

Salt and pepper

**FOR THE SAUCE**
Zest and juice of 1 large orange

2 garlic cloves, minced

1 small teaspoon ginger paste

1 teaspoon toasted sesame oil

4 tablespoons light soy sauce

2 tablespoons rice vinegar

2 tablespoons tomato purée (paste)

2 tablespoons water

Start by preparing all the ingredients, as the cooking process is quick.

Toss the chicken in the cornflour with a pinch each of salt and pepper. Mix the sauce ingredients together in a bowl. In another bowl, toss the cucumber and carrot ribbons with the rice vinegar and coriander. Set aside.

If using uncooked rice, cook according to the packet instructions.

Heat the oil in a large frying pan, add the chicken and stir-fry over a medium heat until lightly browned, about 2 minutes. Add the spring onions and cashews and toss for 2 minutes until the cashews are lightly toasted.

Pour in the sauce and allow to simmer until thickened, about 2–3 minutes.

Serve with the rice, avocado and a handful of cucumber and carrot ribbons.

*I am obsessed with pad Thai. It's a dish I could eat every night. This is my VERY inauthentic version, but I wanted to create something that tasted like the takeaway classic – but with ingredients I can get from my local supermarket that won't cost a fortune.*

# Better-than-takeout Healthy Pad Thai

**SERVES 2**
**Under 360kcal,**
**23g protein per serving**

120g (4oz) dried rice noodles

2 teaspoons toasted sesame oil

Protein of choice (I use 160g/5¾oz prawns/shrimp)

1 garlic clove, minced

2 spring onions (scallions), sliced, plus extra to garnish

1 red (bell) pepper, cored, deseeded and thinly sliced

150g (5½oz) Tenderstem broccoli, spears cut in half

1 carrot, julienned

1 large free-range egg

**FOR THE SAUCE**

1 tablespoon fish sauce

2 tablespoons light soy sauce

1 tablespoon sriracha

Juice of ½ lime

1 small tablespoon tamarind paste

1 tablespoon light brown sugar

1 heaped teaspoon chunky peanut butter

1 tablespoon water

**TO SERVE**

1 lime, cut into wedges

Chopped spring onions (scallions)

Handful of basil leaves

Crushed roasted peanuts (optional)

In a bowl, mix the sauce ingredients together and set aside.

Place the noodles in a large heatproof bowl and pour boiling water over them to cover. Soak for 5 minutes, then drain in a colander and gently rinse under cold water to remove starch. Mix with 1 teaspoon of the sesame oil to keep them from sticking together. They should be al dente and not sticky.

Heat a wok or large frying pan over a high heat with the remaining teaspoon of sesame oil. Brown off your protein, then remove. Add the garlic and vegetables, then toss for 2–3 minutes.

Make space for the egg, add and allow it to set slightly, then scramble. Add the cooked protein, then add the noodles. Pour over the sauce and toss, using a wooden spoon to get any egg off the bottom of the pan. Be gentle when tossing to ensure the noodles do not overcook.

Serve immediately with lime wedges, spring onions, basil and roasted peanuts, if desired.

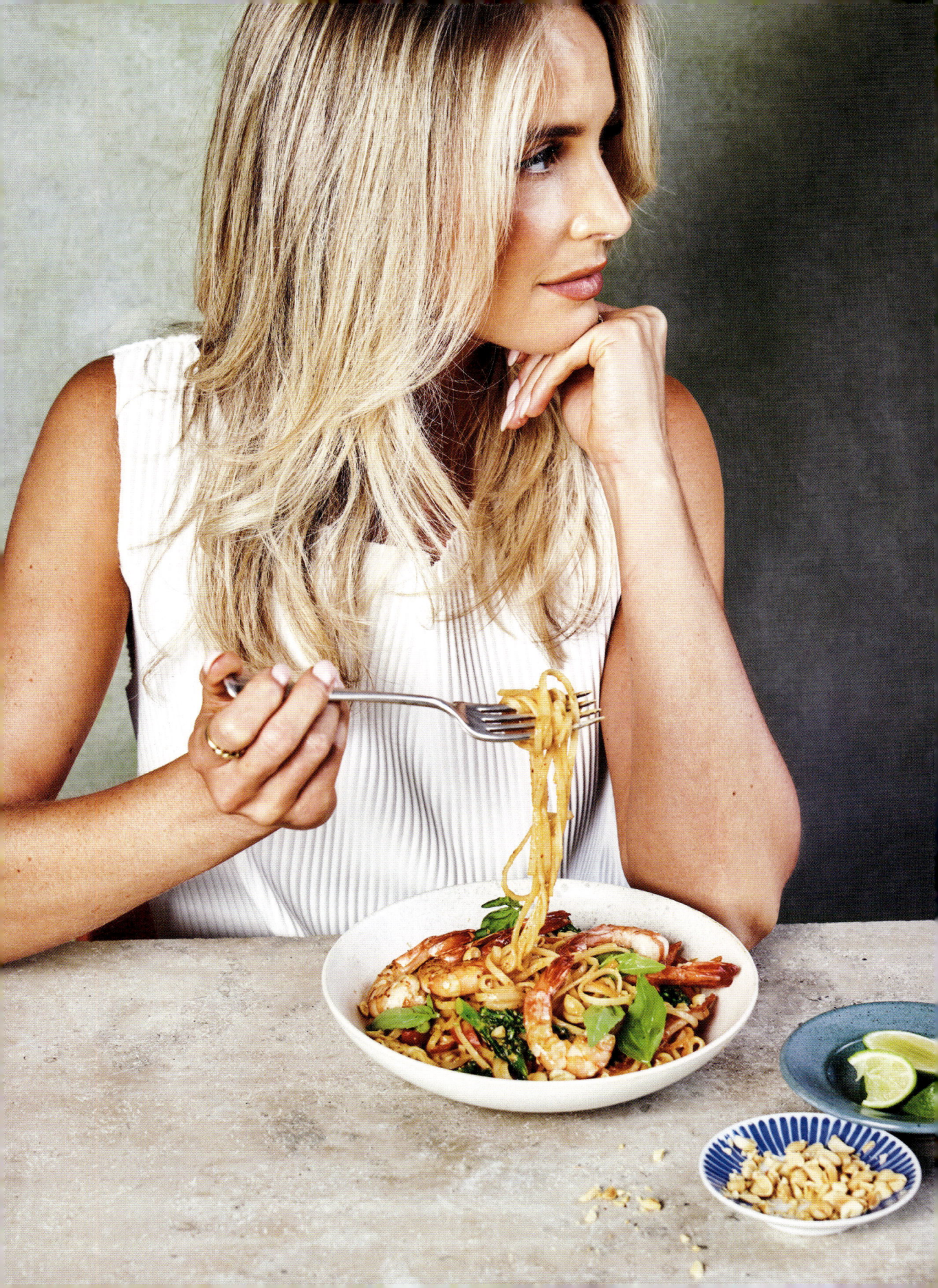

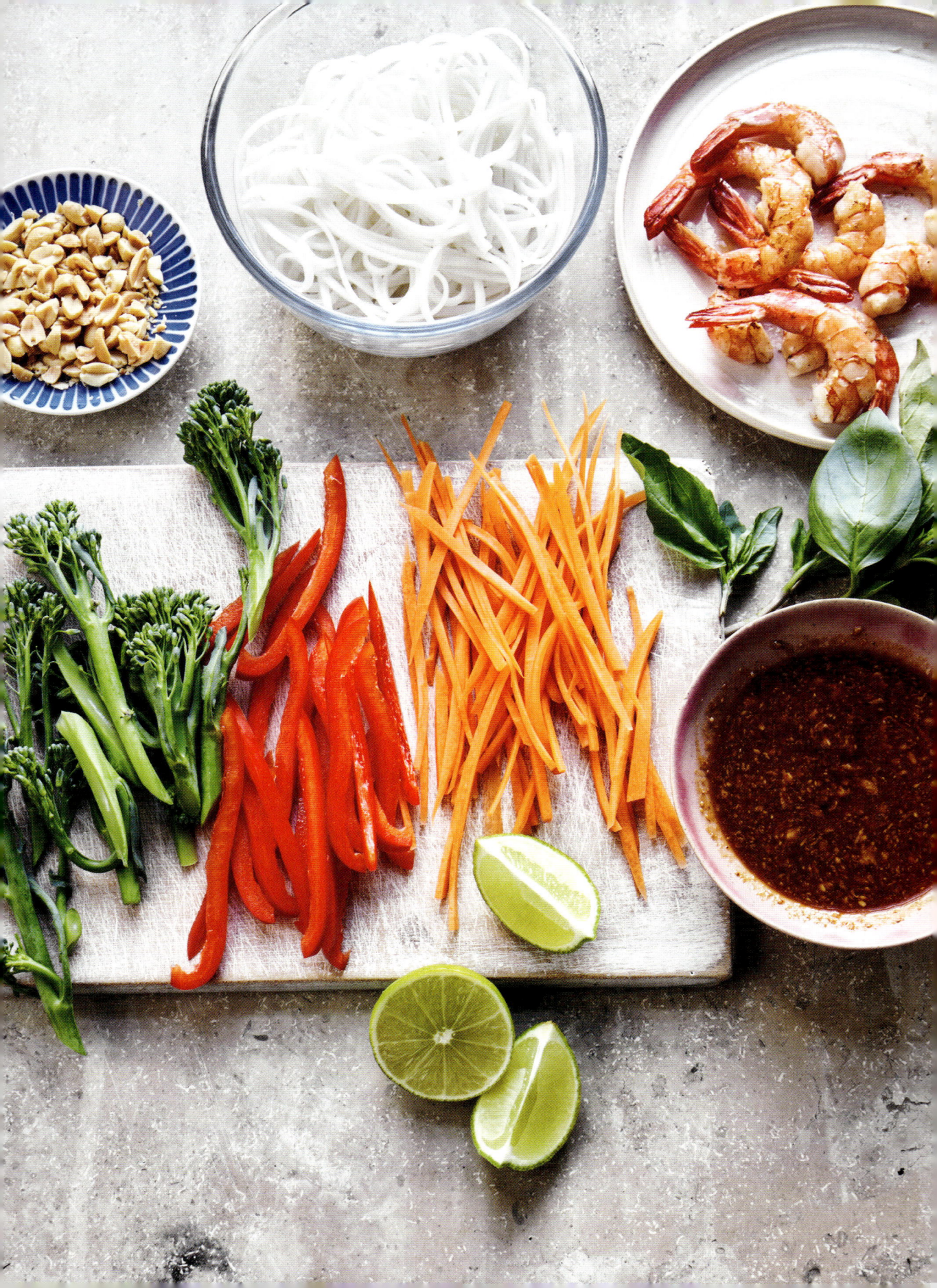

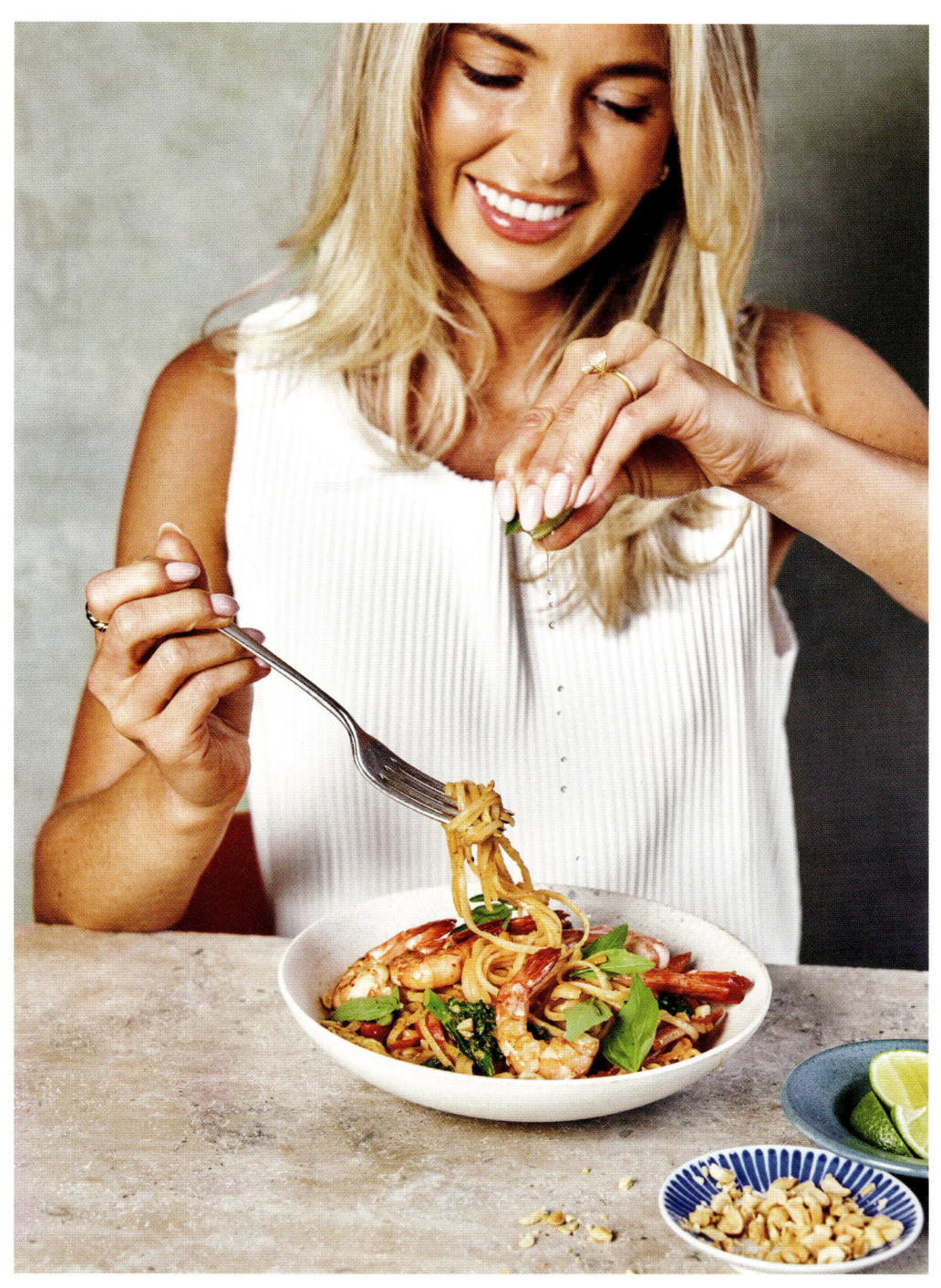

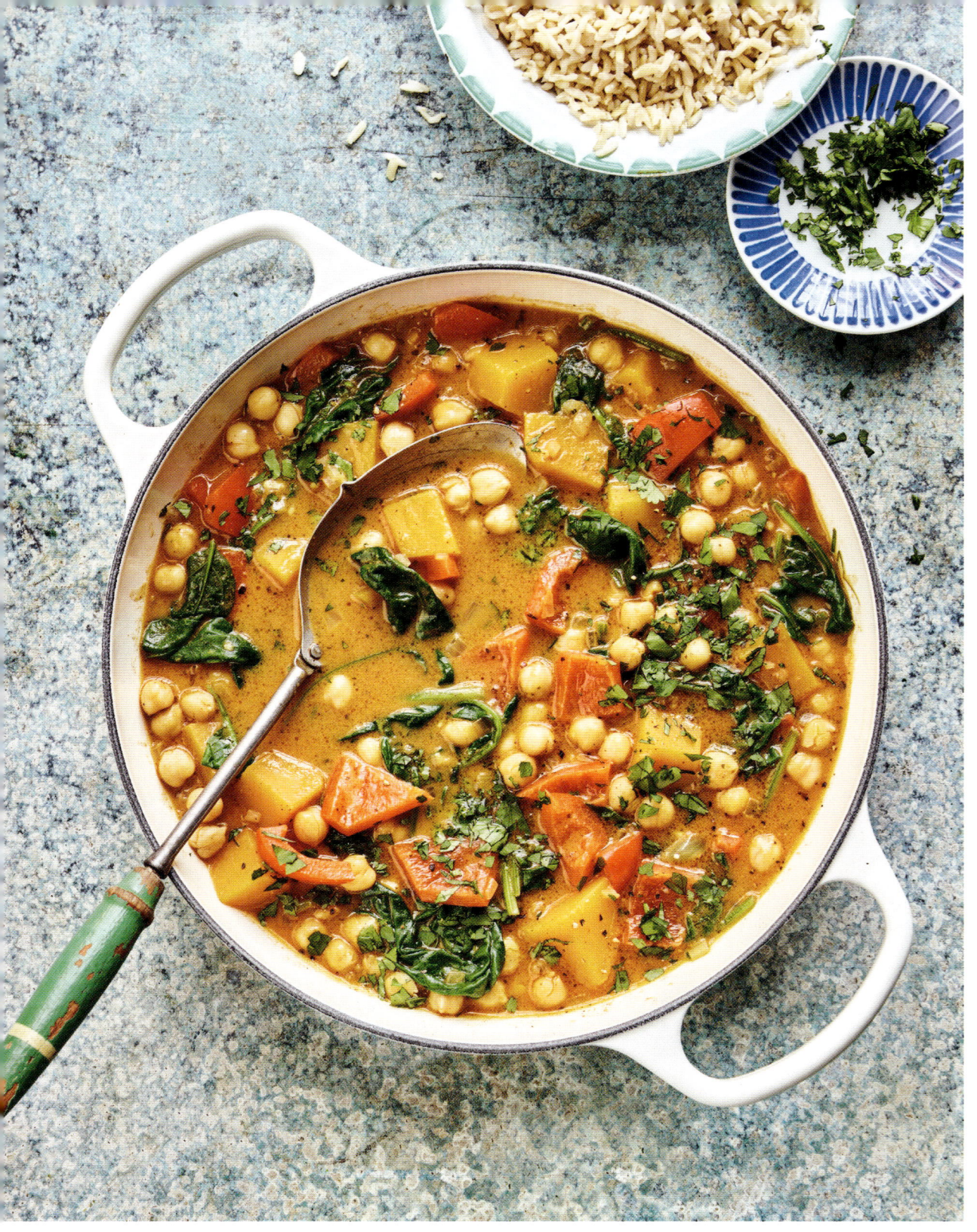

*Creamy, luxurious and perfectly balanced, this is one of my favourite curry recipes. The butternut squash gives it a sweetness and helps it thicken to create the creamiest curry without any cream. It makes the best leftovers and is also freezer-friendly, meaning it's an ideal meal-prep and office-lunch option. I like to incorporate some extra protein, but otherwise this is fully plant-based.*

# Creamy Almond Butter Curry

**SERVES 2**
**Under 640kcal,**
**16g protein per serving**

125g (⅔ cup) brown rice (or use 250g/2 cups precooked rice)

2 teaspoons olive oil, for cooking

1 onion, finely diced

2 garlic cloves, minced

1 heaped tablespoon curry powder

400g (14oz) can of light coconut milk (or regular)

2 generous tablespoons smooth almond butter

1 stock cube (I use chicken), crumbled

1 tablespoon tomato purée (paste)

1 teaspoon honey

1 red (bell) pepper, cored, deseeded and diced

200g (7oz) butternut squash, diced

400g (14oz) can of chickpeas, drained and rinsed

Protein of choice, such as prawns (shrimp), optional (not included in macros)

Handful of baby spinach leaves

Coriander (cilantro) leaves, to garnish

Salt

If cooking your rice from scratch, rinse it in a sieve (strainer) under cold water until the water runs clear. Add the rice to a pan with 250ml (1 cup) water and a pinch of salt. Bring to the boil, then reduce the heat to low, cover and simmer for about 15 minutes until the water is absorbed and the rice is tender. Fluff with a fork before serving.

Meanwhile, heat the olive oil in a deep pan over a low to medium heat, add the onion with a pinch of salt and sweat until softened. Add the garlic and curry powder and cook for another 1–2 minutes. Tip in the coconut milk, fill the can with water and add it to the pan with the almond butter, stock cube, tomato purée and honey. Mix well.

Add the red pepper, squash and chickpeas. Gently simmer for 10 minutes until the squash is soft. If using, add your additional protein, and the spinach, then simmer until cooked.

Serve the curry with the rice and a sprinkle of fresh coriander.

*This one-pan gnocchi dish is a quick and delicious meal that combines the salty richness of Parma ham with the freshness of peas and the creaminess of melted Parmesan. Using the cooking water to create a light yet creamy sauce keeps it healthy and satisfying. Perfect for a busy weeknight dinner.*

# One-pan Pea, Parma Ham and Parmesan Gnocchi

**SERVES 2**
**Under 495kcal,**
**25g protein per serving**

250g (9oz) fresh gnocchi

1 tablespoon olive oil

1 banana shallot, finely diced

2 garlic cloves, minced

4 slices of Parma ham, torn into pieces

150g (1¼ cups) frozen peas, defrosted

2 large handfuls of baby spinach leaves

50g (1¾oz) Parmesan or pecorino cheese, finely grated, plus extra (optional) to serve

Large handful of basil leaves, chopped

Zest of ½ lemon, or more to taste

Salt and pepper

Bring a pan of salted water to the boil, add the gnocchi and cook until they float to the top, about 2–3 minutes. Drain, reserving ½ cup of the cooking water, and set aside.

Heat the olive oil in a large pan over a medium heat. Add the shallot and cook until softened, about 5 minutes. Add the garlic and cook for another minute, until fragrant.

Add the gnocchi to the pan and cook until they start to brown slightly, about 3 minutes. Add the Parma ham and peas and cook for another 5 minutes until the ham starts to crisp and the peas are heated through. Add the spinach and cook until wilted, about 1–2 minutes.

Add 100ml (scant ½ cup) of the reserved cooking water and scatter the grated cheese evenly over the gnocchi mixture. Allow 30 seconds for the cheese to melt, then toss everything well and stir together to make a smooth, shiny sauce. If needed, add a splash more cooking water to loosen the sauce further and coat the gnocchi.

Season with salt and lots of pepper to taste. Continue to toss for another 2–3 minutes until the sauce has thickened and is coating the gnocchi. Stir in the basil and lemon zest.

Serve immediately, topped with extra cheese if desired.

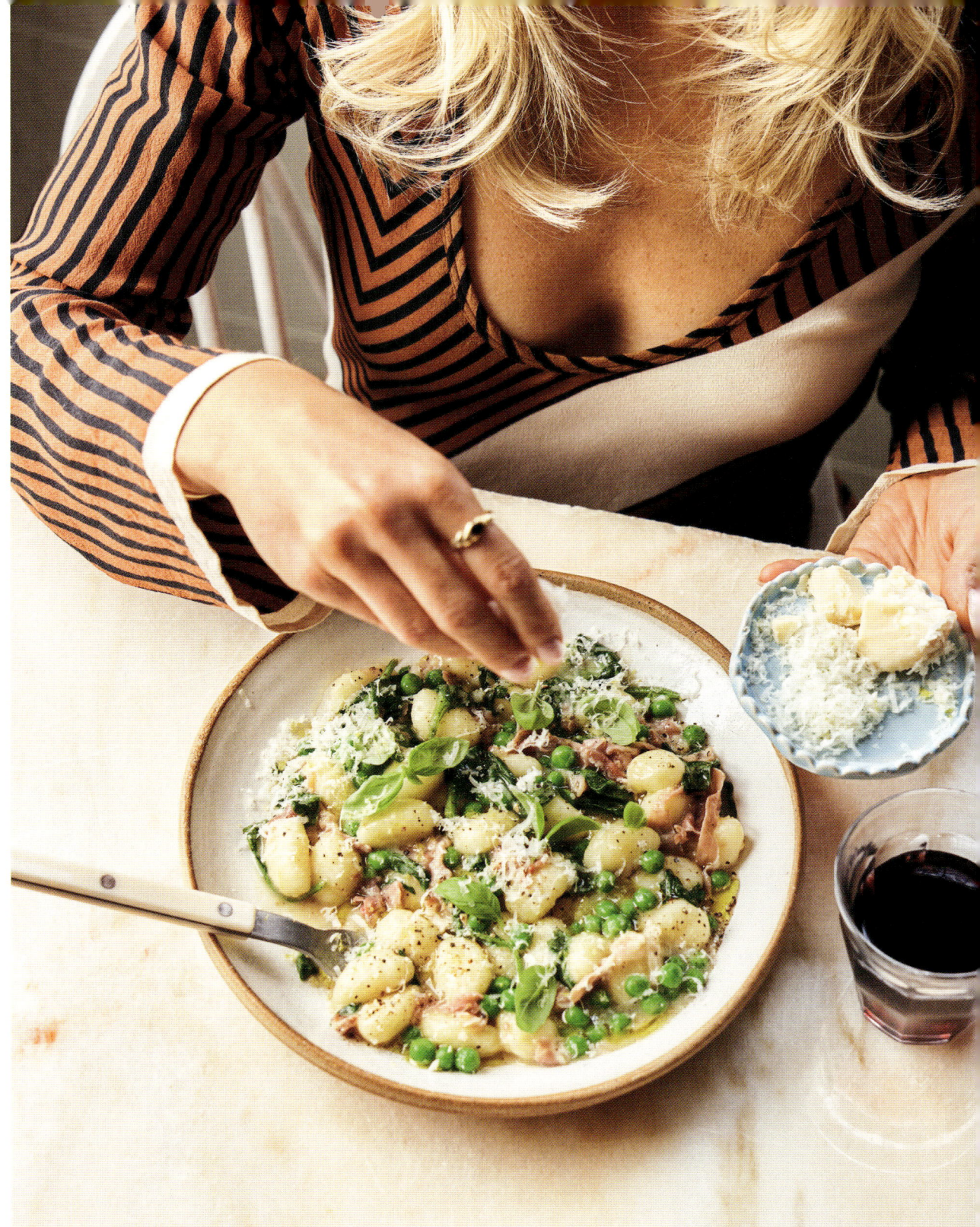

*This is a meal I make when I'm busy or tired. It's all in one pot, uses only a few ingredients and comes together in 30 minutes. Leftovers also heat up like a dream, and I eat them for lunch the next day. You can pair this with any protein you like; it's very versatile. I also love to have an extra side of greens!*

# Easy One-pot Creamy Mushroom Risotto

**SERVES 2**
**Under 300kcal,**
**12g protein per serving**

300g (10½oz) chestnut
    mushrooms
1 teaspoon olive oil
1 onion, diced
2 large garlic cloves, diced
1 teaspoon chopped
    rosemary leaves
140g (¾ cup) risotto rice
    (Arborio or Carnaroli)
1 tablespoon porcini
    mushroom paste
1 teaspoon white miso
500ml (generous 2 cups) water
1 chicken or veg stock
    cube, crumbled
50g (1¾oz) Parmesan cheese,
    grated, and its rind
1 tablespoon half-fat
    crème fraîche
1 teaspoon honey (truffle
    honey if you have it)
Salt and pepper

**TO SERVE**
Protein of choice
1 tablespoon chopped chives

Chop the mushrooms into different sizes to add texture – some big and some small.

Heat the olive oil in a deep pan over a low to medium heat, add the onion and sweat for a minute or so. Add the mushrooms, garlic, rosemary and a few cracks of pepper (no salt yet). Cook for 10 minutes until all the water comes from the mushrooms and evaporates. Now season with salt.

Add the rice, porcini paste and miso, stir for a minute, then tip in 300ml (1¼ cups) of the water, the stock cube and Parmesan rind.

Allow to simmer gently, mixing from time to time to prevent the rice from sticking to the bottom of the pan and to help it thicken. Gradually add more of the water, stirring frequently, until the rice is al dente and creamy, about 18–20 minutes.

Whisk in the crème fraîche, honey, grated Parmesan, and some extra pepper or salt if needed. Serve with your protein of choice and a scattering of chopped chives.

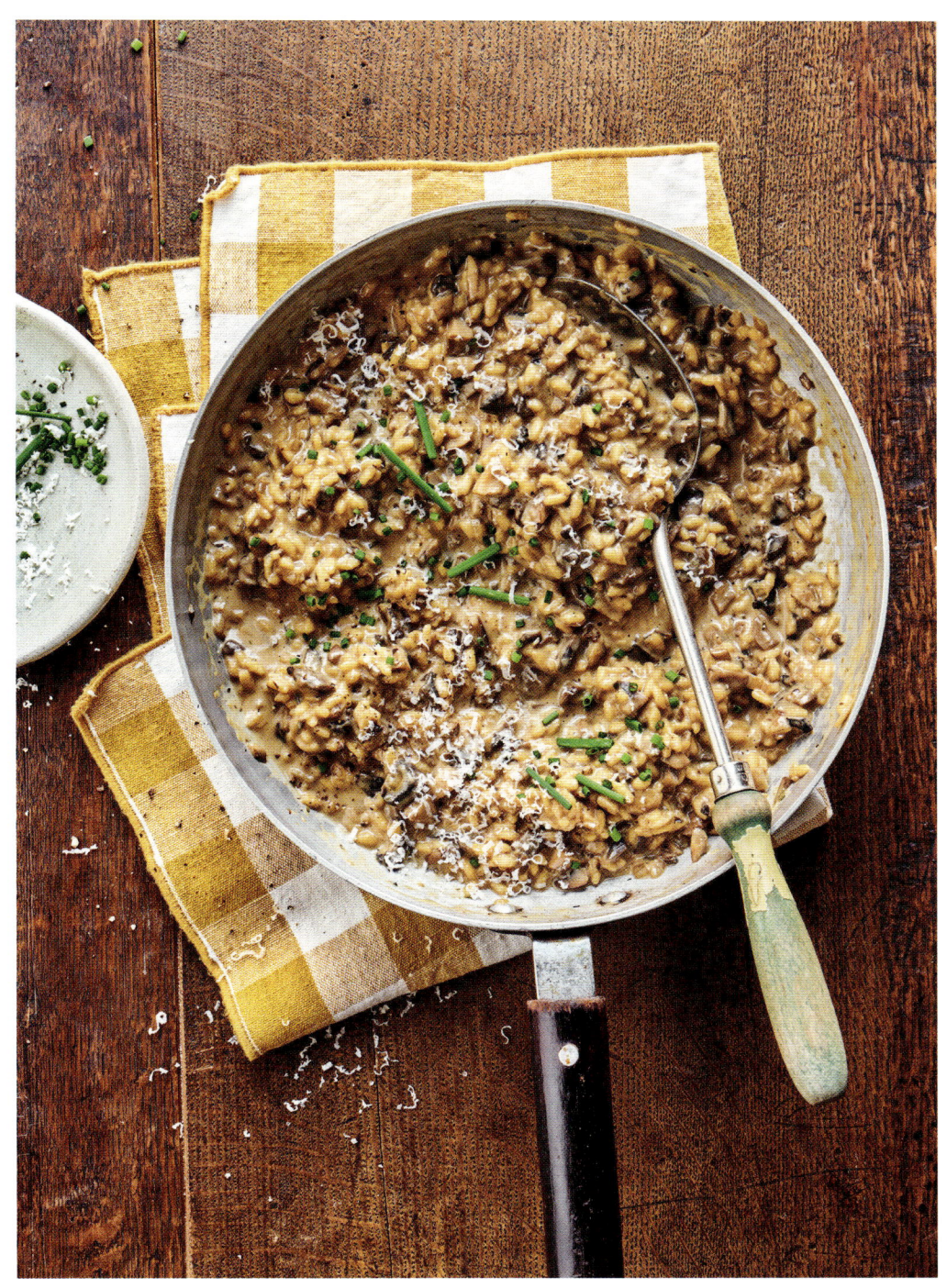

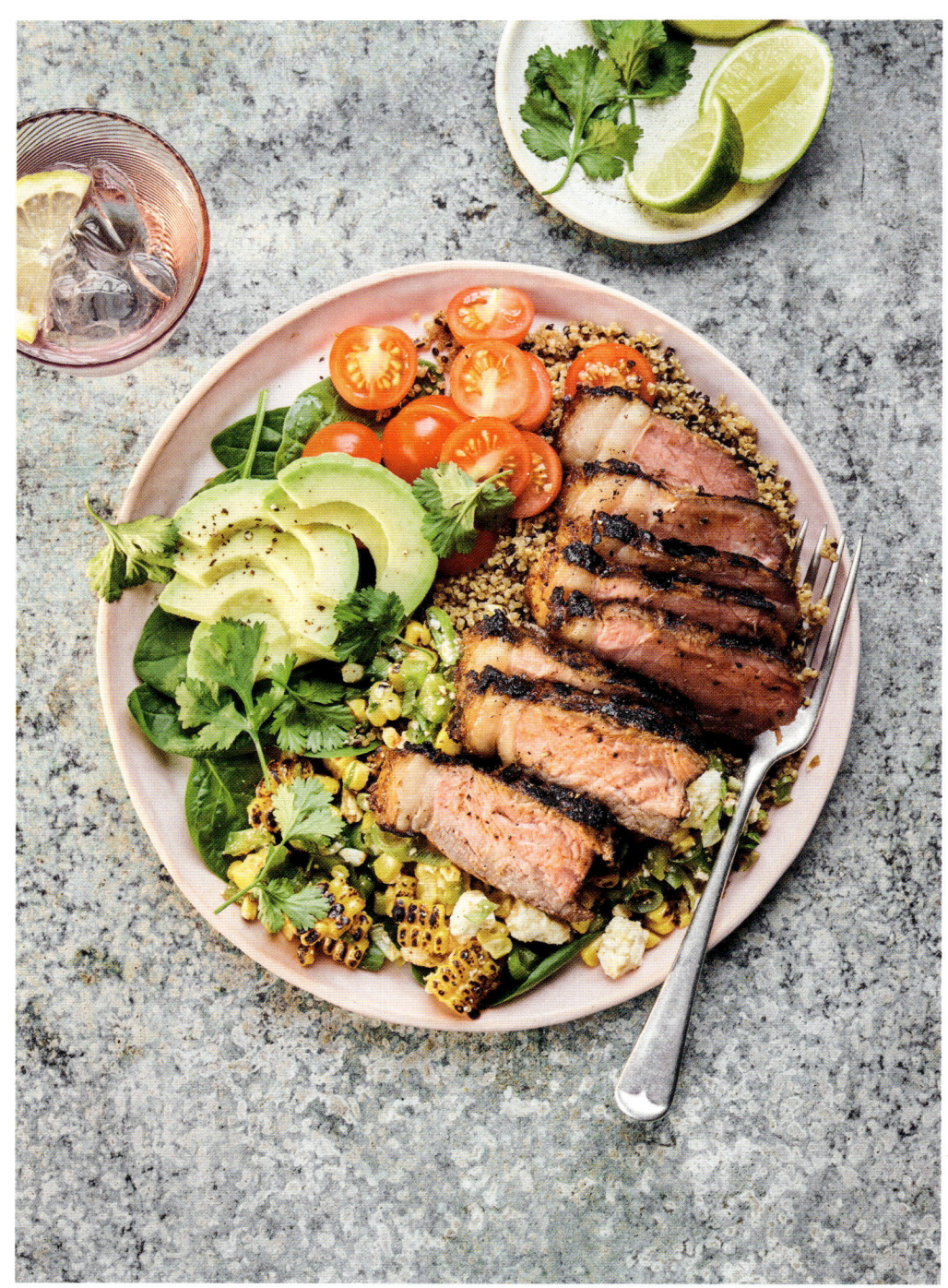

*Seared chipotle steak bowls full of punchy spice, a creamy corn salad and lots of fresh zippy lime. I love a good wellness bowl, which is one of my favourite ways to enjoy a good steak. A satisfying yet healthy recipe.*

# Seared Chipotle Steak Bowls with Charred Corn Salad

**SERVES 2**
**Under 870kcal,**
**62g protein per serving**

1 tablespoon chipotle paste

1 tablespoon olive oil

1 garlic clove, minced

Juice of 1 lime

350–400g (12–14oz) sirloin steak (or use any steak you like)

Handful of baby spinach leaves

250g (9oz) cooked quinoa or brown rice, to serve (optional)

½ medium ripe avocado, peeled, pitted and sliced

Handful of cherry tomatoes, halved

Salt and pepper

Lime wedges, to serve

**FOR THE CHARRED CORN SALAD**

2 ears of corn, husked

3 spring onions (scallions), finely chopped

1 green (bell) pepper, cored, deseeded and chopped

Handful of coriander (cilantro) leaves, chopped, plus extra (optional) to serve

80g (2¾oz) feta cheese, crumbled

1 heaped tablespoon Greek yogurt (0% or full fat)

Juice of 1 lime

1 teaspoon smoked paprika

1 tablespoon chopped jalapeños from a jar, plus 1 tablespoon of the brine

1 heaped teaspoon honey

Few dashes of Tabasco

Mix the chipotle paste, olive oil, garlic and lime juice with some salt and pepper in a small bowl. Rub the mixture all over the steak and let it marinate for at least 30 minutes, preferably longer.

For the charred corn salad, heat a grill pan over medium-high heat. Grill (broil) the corn until charred on all sides, about 8–10 minutes. Remove from the heat and let cool slightly. Cut the kernels off the cob and place them in a large bowl. Add the spring onions, green pepper, coriander and feta. Mix in the yogurt, lime juice, smoked paprika, jalapeños and brine, honey and Tabasco, with salt and pepper to taste, and toss to combine.

Heat a large frying pan over a medium-high heat. Sear the steak for 3 minutes on each side for medium-rare, or until cooked to your desired level of doneness. Remove from the frying pan and let it rest for 5 minutes before slicing.

Divide the baby spinach between the bases of 2 bowls. Add the cooked quinoa or rice, if using. Top with the avocado, tomatoes and charred corn salad. Add the sliced steak on top and garnish with lime wedges, and extra coriander, if desired.

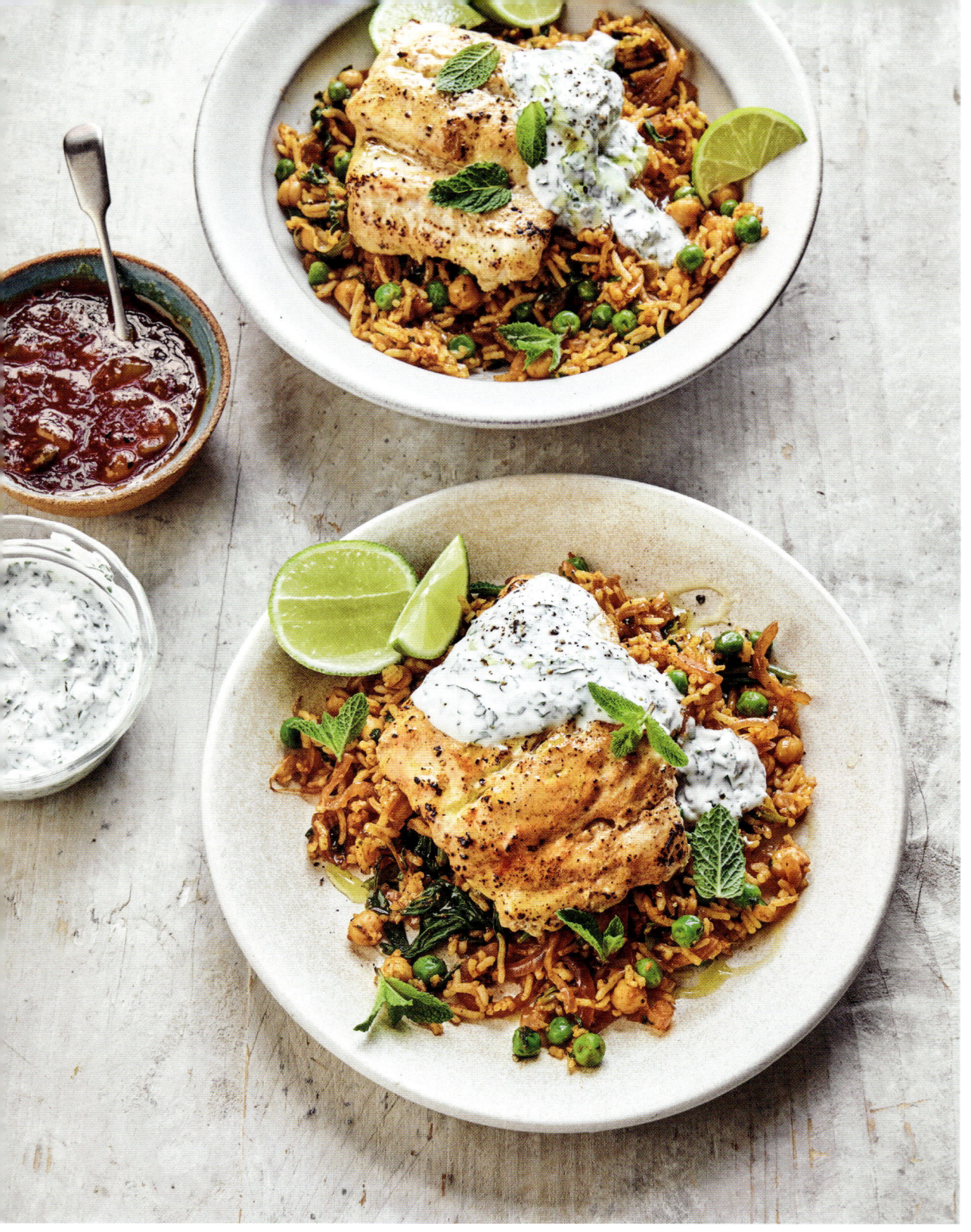

*This is one of my favourite recipes I have created to date, combining the rich, spiced flavours of tikka-marinated cod with the sweetness of caramelised onions, using a touch of mango chutney. Aromatic, fragrant and simple to make. Paired with a refreshing mint raita, this is a dish I eat all year round.*

# Tikka Cod with Caramelised Onion Rice

**SERVES 2**
**Under 693kcal,**
**44g protein per serving**

2 skinless cod fillets
Salt and pepper

**FOR THE MARINADE**
2 tablespoons Greek
  yogurt (ideally full fat)
Juice of 1 lemon
1 teaspoon ginger paste
1 teaspoon garlic paste
1 teaspoon garam masala
1 teaspoon mango chutney
1 teaspoon tomato
  purée (paste)

**FOR THE CARAMELISED**
**ONION RICE**
2 teaspoons olive oil
2 red onions, finely sliced
1 tablespoon mango chutney
1 tablespoon garam masala
1 tablespoon tomato
  purée (paste)
80g (½ cup) frozen peas
½ x 400g (14oz) can of
  chickpeas, drained
  and rinsed
250g (2 cups) precooked rice
Handful of baby
  spinach leaves

**FOR THE RAITA**
150g (⅔ cup) Greek yogurt
  (ideally full fat)
2 tablespoons chopped
  coriander (cilantro) leaves
1 tablespoon chopped
  mint leaves
Juice of ½ lemon

In a small bowl, mix together the marinade ingredients, with salt and pepper to taste. Coat the cod fillets in the marinade and let them sit for at least 30 minutes.

Preheat the oven to 220°C/200°C fan (425°F) Gas Mark 7, or the air fryer to 200°C (400°F).

In a large pan, heat the olive oil over a medium heat. Add the red onions and mango chutney and cook until caramelised, about 10–15 minutes, adding a splash of water if they start to catch on the bottom of the pan. Stir in the garam masala and tomato purée and cook for another 2 minutes until aromatic.

Add the frozen peas and chickpeas and sauté for about 3 minutes, until everything is heated, then add the precooked rice and spinach, mix until coated and cook for a final few minutes until the rice is hot and the spinach wilted.

Place the marinated cod fillets on a baking sheet and bake in the oven for 10–15 minutes, or in the air fryer for 12–15 minutes, until cooked through and the cod flakes easily with a fork.

Meanwhile, mix the raita ingredients, with salt and pepper to taste, in a small bowl.

Place a generous portion of the caramelised onion rice on each plate. Top with the cod fillet and a dollop of mint raita. Serve with a side of greens, if desired.

*Prawn saganaki is one of my favourite things to eat in Greece. This is my hybrid of those flavours but in a one-pot orzo form. It makes great meal prep and heats up really well too. If you don't like prawns, substitute them for any protein you like.*

# Prawn Saganaki Orzo

**SERVES 2**
**Under 515kcal,**
**32.5g protein per serving**

1 tablespoon olive oil
3 garlic cloves, minced
2 shallots, finely chopped
1 red chilli, finely chopped
(deseeded if you like)
1 red (bell) pepper,
deseeded and diced
200g (7oz) cherry
tomatoes, halved
400g (14oz) can of
chopped tomatoes
150g (5½oz) orzo
1 chicken (or veg) stock cube
1 teaspoon dried oregano
60g (2¼oz) spinach,
roughly chopped
Zest and juice of 1 lemon
200g (7oz) raw prawns
(shrimp), peeled
and deveined
Salt and pepper

**TO SERVE**
80g (2¾oz) feta cheese,
crumbled
Fresh dill and parsley leaves

Heat the olive oil in a large pan over a medium heat. Add the garlic, shallots and chilli and sauté for 2–3 minutes, until fragrant and translucent.

Add the red pepper and cook for about 5 minutes, until softened. Add the cherry tomatoes and cook until they start to soften and release their juices, about 3–4 minutes.

Stir in the canned tomatoes, then half-fill the empty can with water and add this too. Add the orzo, stock cube and oregano, and season with salt and pepper. Let it simmer for about 15 minutes until the orzo is cooked, topping up with a splash of water if needed and stirring often to stop the orzo sticking.

Stir in the spinach and the lemon zest and juice. Once the spinach has wilted, gently fold in the prawns. Allow to simmer gently for 5 minutes to cook the prawns through. Sprinkle the crumbled feta and fresh herbs over the top to serve.

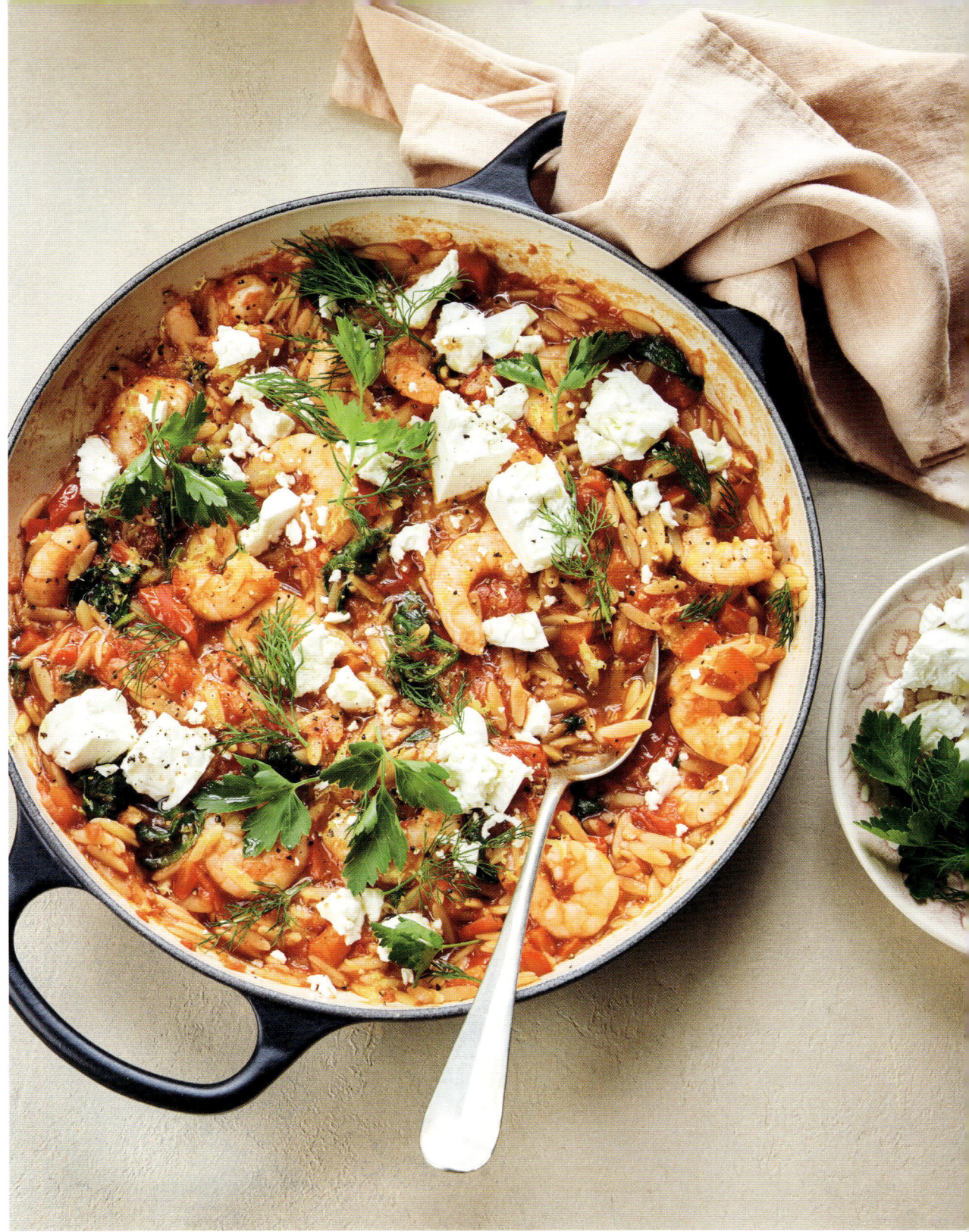

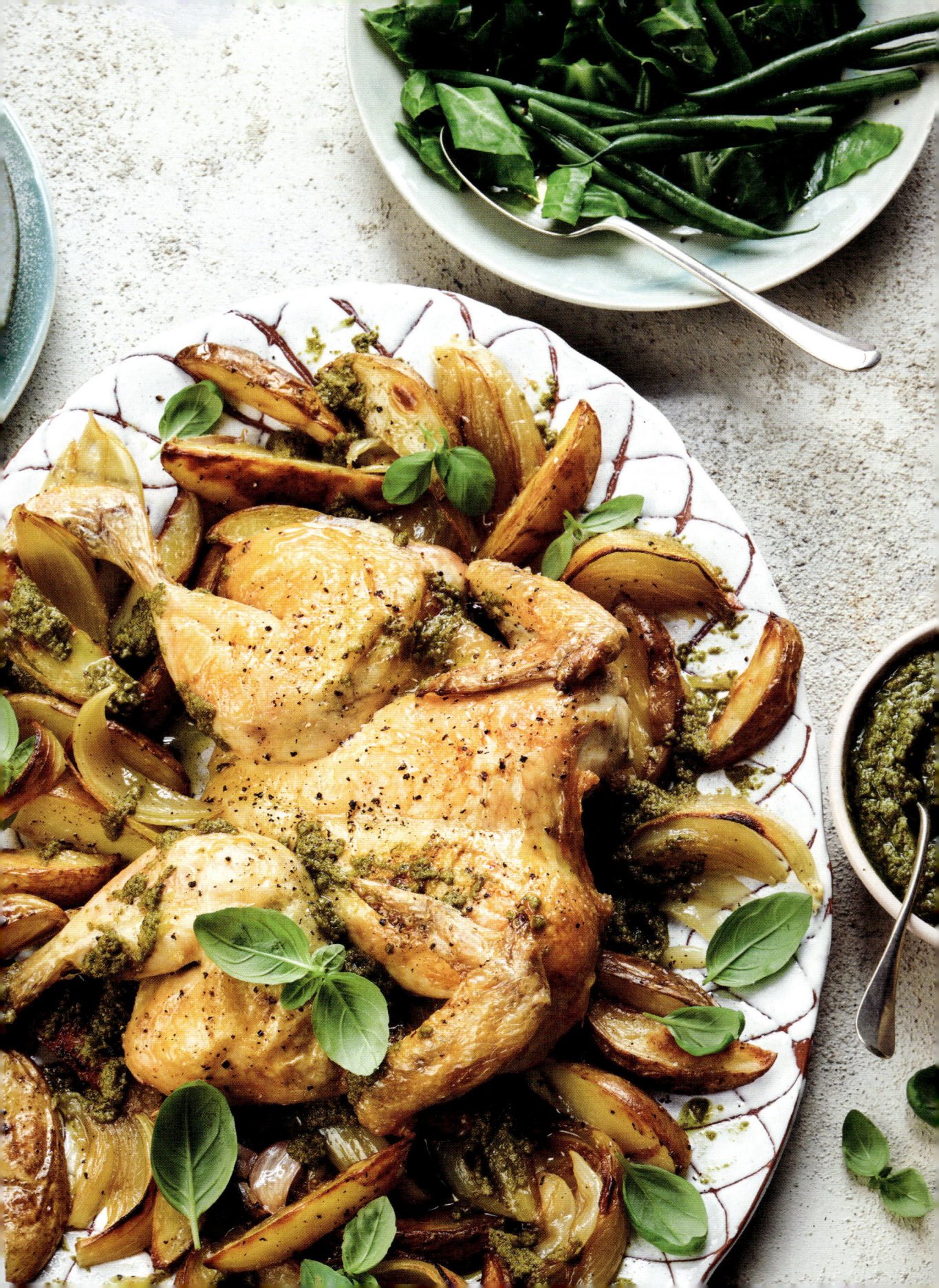

*This wonderful roast chicken recipe is paired with a delicious homemade pesto with lots of fresh rosemary and toasted hazelnuts. It's the perfect recipe for when you want a lighter, low-effort roast dinner.*

# Spatchcock Chicken with Rosemary Pesto

**SERVES 4**
**Under 545kcal,**
**48g protein per serving**

1 medium whole chicken

4 garlic cloves, smashed with skin on

2 onions, cut into wedges

700g (1lb 9oz) potatoes, cut into wedges

Mild extra virgin olive oil

Salt and pepper

300g (10½oz) cooked green beans, to serve

**FOR THE ROSEMARY PESTO**

60g (½ cup) skin-on hazelnuts

30g (¼ cup) skin-on almonds

2 sprigs of rosemary, leaves stripped

30g (1oz) basil leaves

50g (1¾oz) Parmesan cheese, grated

1 garlic clove, roughly chopped

Zest and juice of 1 lemon

100ml (3½fl oz) mild extra virgin olive oil

Preheat the oven to 180°C/160°C fan (350°F) Gas Mark 4. Spread the hazelnuts and almonds on a baking sheet and toast in the oven for 5–7 minutes, until fragrant. Remove and set aside to cool slightly. Increase the oven temperature to 200°C/180°C fan (400°F) Gas Mark 6.

To spatchcock the chicken, place the chicken breast-side down on a chopping board. Using kitchen shears, cut along both sides of the backbone and remove it. Flip the chicken over and press down firmly on the breastbone to flatten.

On a large baking tray, arrange the spatchcocked chicken, garlic cloves, onion and potato wedges. Drizzle everything with olive oil and season with salt and pepper. Toss the onions and potatoes in the oil to coat evenly, transfer to the oven and roast for 45–50 minutes, or until the chicken is cooked through and the potatoes are golden and tender. The internal temperature of the chicken should reach 75°C (165°F).

Meanwhile, heat 1 tablespoon of olive oil in a small pan over a medium heat. Once hot, add the rosemary leaves and fry until crispy, about 1 minute. Remove the leaves and set them on kitchen paper to drain.

In a food processor, combine the toasted hazelnuts, almonds, basil, crispy rosemary, Parmesan, garlic and the lemon zest and juice. Pulse until finely chopped. With the processor running, gradually pour in enough olive oil until a smooth, thick pesto forms. If needed, add more olive oil or a bit of water to reach the desired consistency. Season with salt and pepper to taste.

Transfer the roasted chicken and vegetables to a serving platter. Serve with a drizzle of the rosemary pesto on the side, and some green beans.

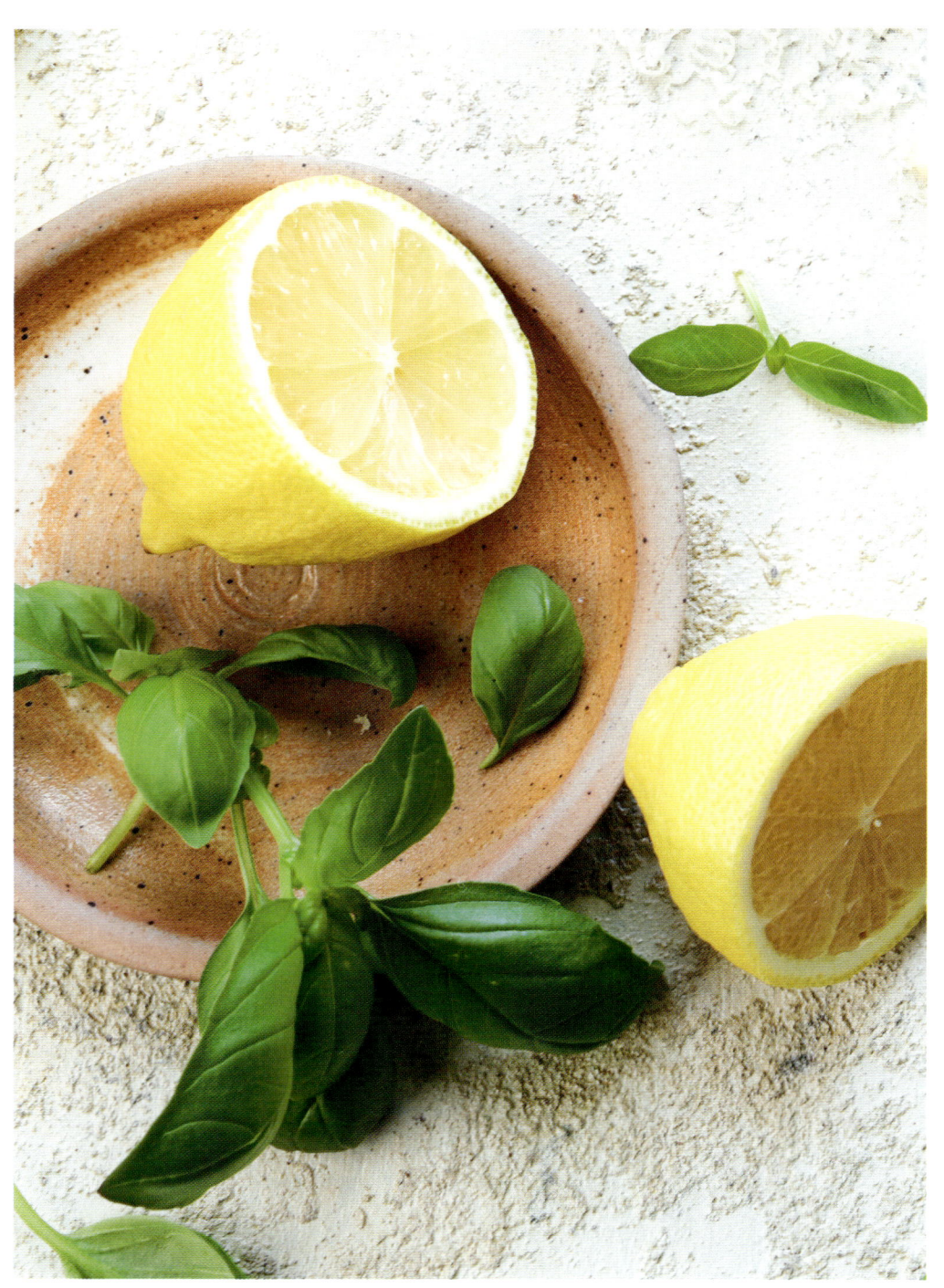

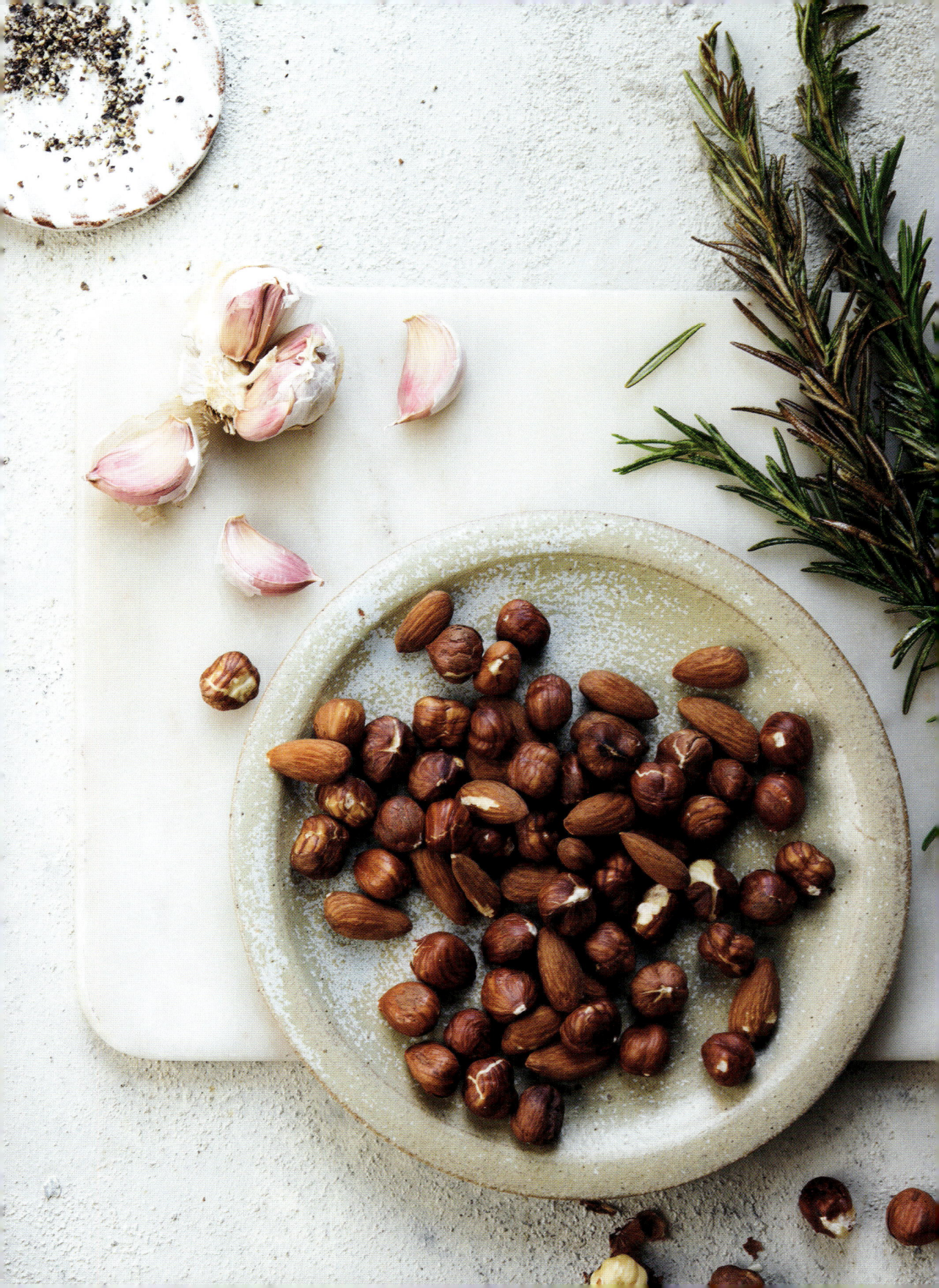

*A combination of crushed baby potatoes mixed with a savoury pipérade, which consists of red peppers, onions, olives and garlic seasoned with sweet smoked paprika. I serve it here with crispy-skin sea bass and a simple dollop of garlic yogurt. The perfect dinner makes great leftovers too. Use any protein you like instead of sea bass, to suit your preferences.*

# Crushed Pipérade Potatoes with Garlic Yogurt and Sea Bass

**SERVES 2**
**Under 500kcal,**
**34g protein per serving**

Olive oil, for cooking
2 sea bass fillets (skin on)
Salt and pepper
Squeeze of lemon
    juice, to serve

**FOR THE PIPÉRADE POTATOES**
400g (14oz) waxy baby
    potatoes, such as Jersey
    Royals (skin on)
1 large red onion, finely sliced
1 red (bell) pepper, cored,
    deseeded and finely sliced
1 yellow (bell) pepper, cored,
    deseeded and finely sliced
2 garlic cloves, roughly
    chopped
2 heaped teaspoons sweet
    smoked paprika
1 tablespoon tomato
    purée (paste)
3 vine-ripened tomatoes,
    roughly chopped
12 pitted Kalamata
    olives, halved
2 tablespoons finely chopped
    parsley, plus extra to garnish

**FOR THE GARLIC YOGURT**
100g (scant ½ cup) thick
    Greek yogurt
½ garlic clove, minced
Zest of ½ lemon

Bring a pan of salted water to the boil. Add the potatoes and cook until tender, about 15 minutes. Drain and very lightly press the potatoes with the back of a serving spoon, leaving them chunky but bursting. Set aside.

While the potatoes are cooking, heat 1 tablespoon of olive oil in a pan over a medium heat. Add the red onion and peppers and cook until softened, about 10 minutes.

Add the garlic and smoked paprika, cooking for another 2 minutes until fragrant. Stir in the tomato purée and tomatoes. Cook for an additional 5 minutes until the tomatoes begin to break down and form a sauce. Add the olives and cook for another 2 minutes. Season with salt and pepper to taste, then combine the pipérade mixture with the crushed potatoes and mix gently. Stir in the chopped parsley.

For the garlic yogurt, combine the yogurt, garlic, lemon zest and salt and pepper to taste in a small bowl. Mix well and set aside.

Dry and season the sea bass fillets with salt and pepper. Heat 2 teaspoons of olive oil in a large nonstick frying pan over medium-high heat. Place the sea bass fillets skin-side down and cook for 3–4 minutes until the skin is crispy. Flip the fillets and immediately take off the heat. Let sit for 30 seconds, then remove.

To serve, spoon the pipérade potatoes on to plates. Place the sea bass on top and add a dollop of garlic yogurt. Garnish with parsley and a squeeze of lemon.

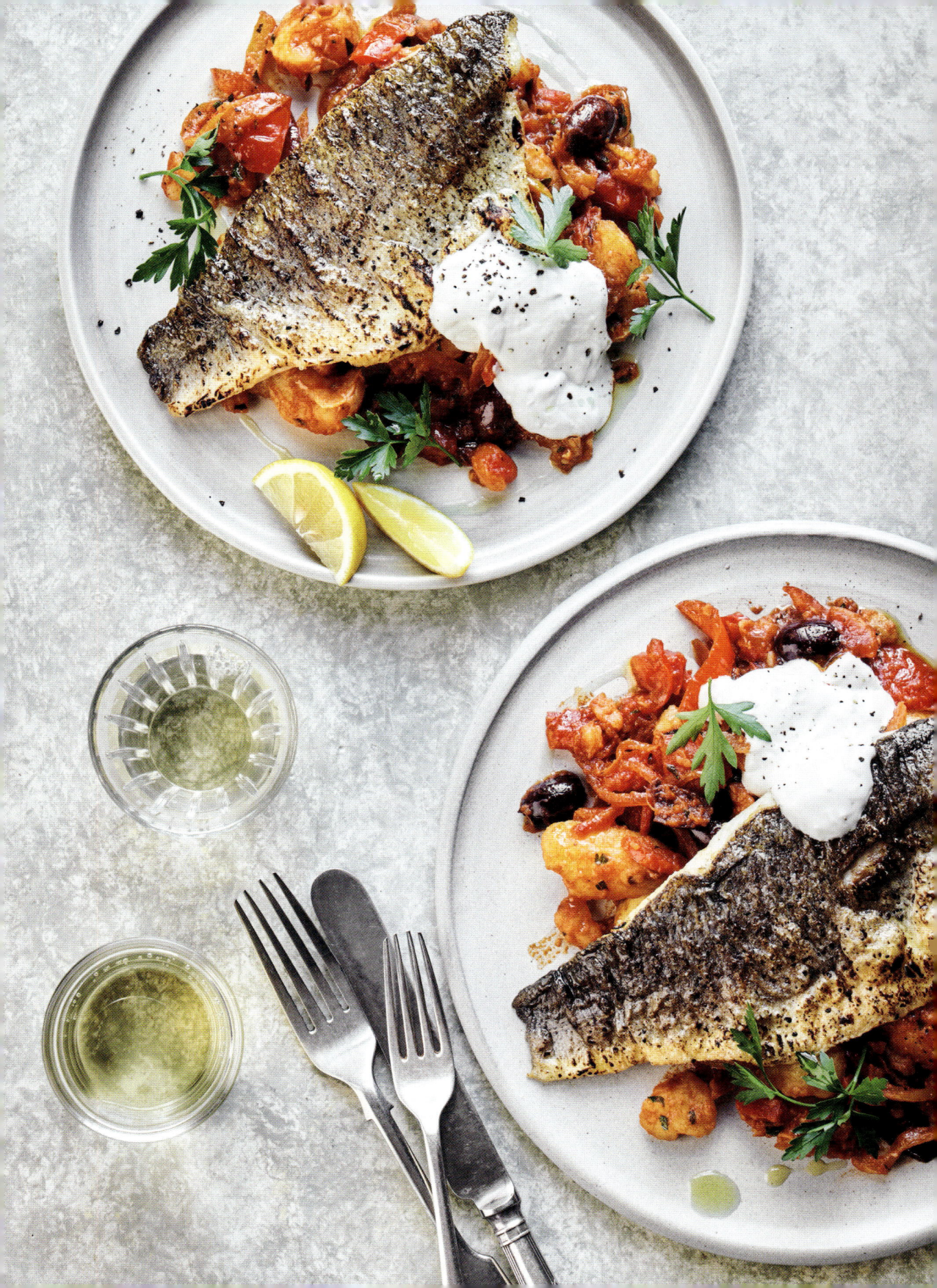

# Sweet

Peanut Butter and Jam Blondies | *Greek Yogurt and Honey Panna Cotta with Fresh Raspberries* | Dark Chocolate Orange Silken Tofu Pots | *Layered Spiced Apple Cake* | Strawberry Shortcake Yogurt Breakfast Loaf | *Carrot Cake with Maple Cream Cheese Frosting* | Mango Upside-down Cake with Almond, Yogurt and Miso Caramel | *Granny's Hazelnut Meringues with Light Coffee Cream* | Toasted Oat Chocolate Tiffin | *Instant Frozen Berry Yogurt*

*These delicious chickpea blondies will convert any healthy-baking sceptic. They are perfect for a healthier dessert option, with some protein and good-for-you ingredients. The texture is fudgy, and the chickpeas add a nutty taste that works so well.*

# Peanut Butter and Jam Blondies

**MAKES 12 SQUARES**
**Under 130kcal,**
**5g protein per serving**

400g (14oz) can of chickpeas, drained, rinsed and dried

80g (⅓ cup) smooth peanut butter

120ml (½ cup) maple syrup or honey

1 teaspoon vanilla extract

½ teaspoon baking powder

½ teaspoon bicarbonate of soda (baking soda)

Pinch of salt

3 heaped tablespoons ground almonds

3 heaped tablespoons rolled oats

Handful of raspberries

Handful of flaked (slivered) almonds

Preheat the oven to 190°C/170°C fan (375°F) Gas Mark 5.

Combine the chickpeas with the peanut butter, maple syrup or honey, vanilla extract, baking powder, bicarb, salt, ground almonds and oats in a blender and blend until smooth. Avoid over-mixing.

Pour the mixture into a 20cm (8 inch) square nonstick baking tin (pan). Sprinkle the fresh raspberries and flaked almonds on top.

Bake for 30–35 minutes or until a toothpick inserted into the centre comes out clean. Allow to cool slightly to firm up, then slice into squares and enjoy.

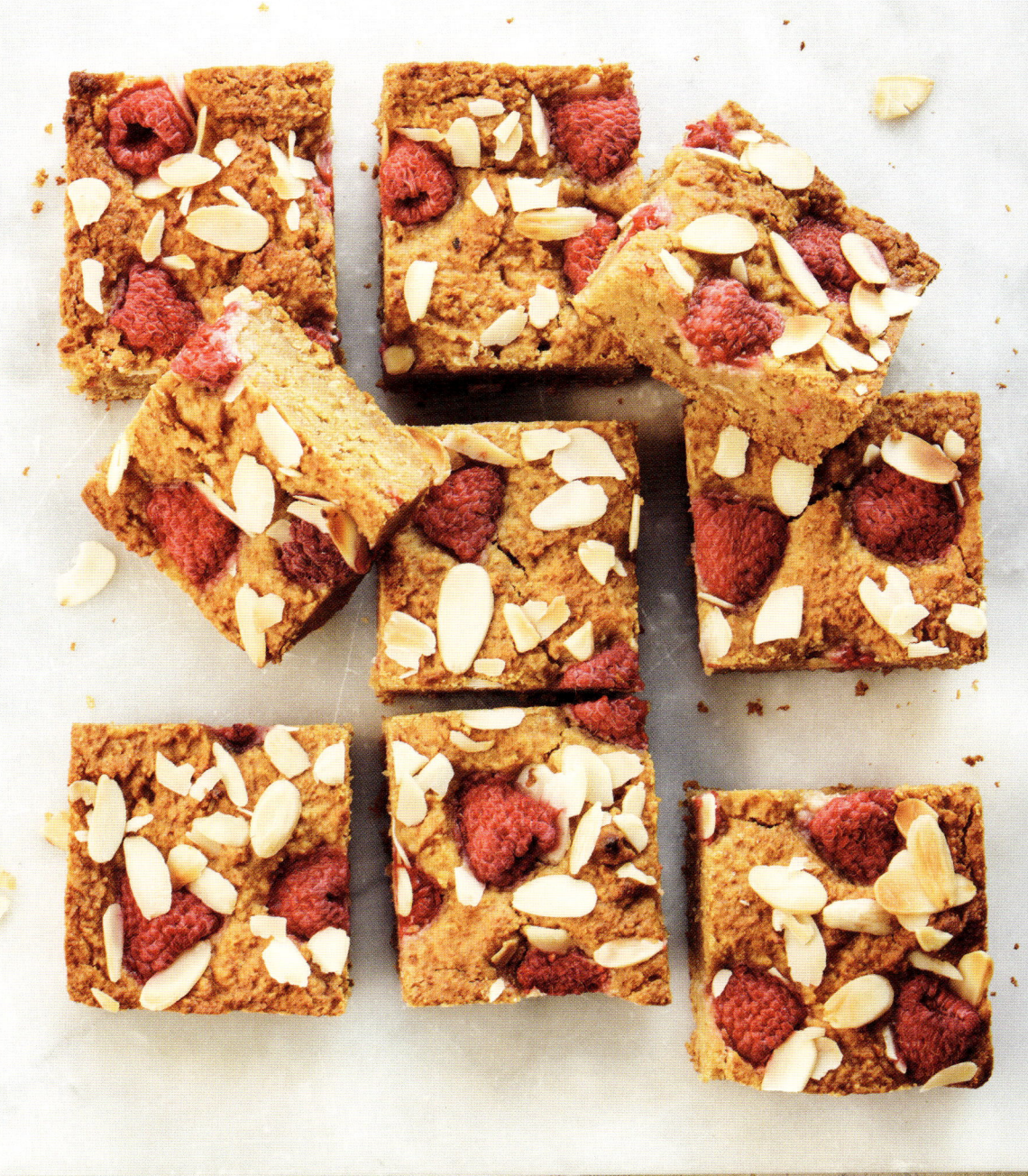

*This panna cotta is a light and creamy dessert that perfectly balances the tanginess of the yogurt with the sweetness of the honey. It has the silky texture of an indulgent dessert. Pair with fresh raspberries to serve.*

# Greek Yogurt and Honey Panna Cotta with Fresh Raspberries

**SERVES 4**
**Under 340kcal,**
**18g protein per serving**

4½ sheets of leaf gelatine
200ml (scant 1 cup)
    single (light) cream
200ml (scant 1 cup) whole milk
1 teaspoon high-quality
    vanilla paste
100g (⅓ cup) honey
500g (generous 2 cups)
    full-fat Greek yogurt
Raspberries, to serve

Submerge the gelatine in a bowl of cold water for 5–10 minutes to soften.

Put the cream, milk, vanilla paste and honey into a pan. Place over a medium-low heat until the mixture starts to bubble, then take off the heat.

When the cream has settled to being just warm to the touch, drain the gelatine, squeezing out excess water, and stir into the cream until it has completely dissolved. Add the yogurt and whisk until smooth and combined, then strain the mixture to remove any lumps.

Divide the mixture between 4 small glasses, moulds or espresso cups. Place on a tray lined with kitchen paper to prevent them from sliding around. Cool, cover and refrigerate overnight to set.

Run a knife around the edges of each panna cotta and carefully invert it on to a plate, or serve directly in the cups or glasses, topped with fresh raspberries.

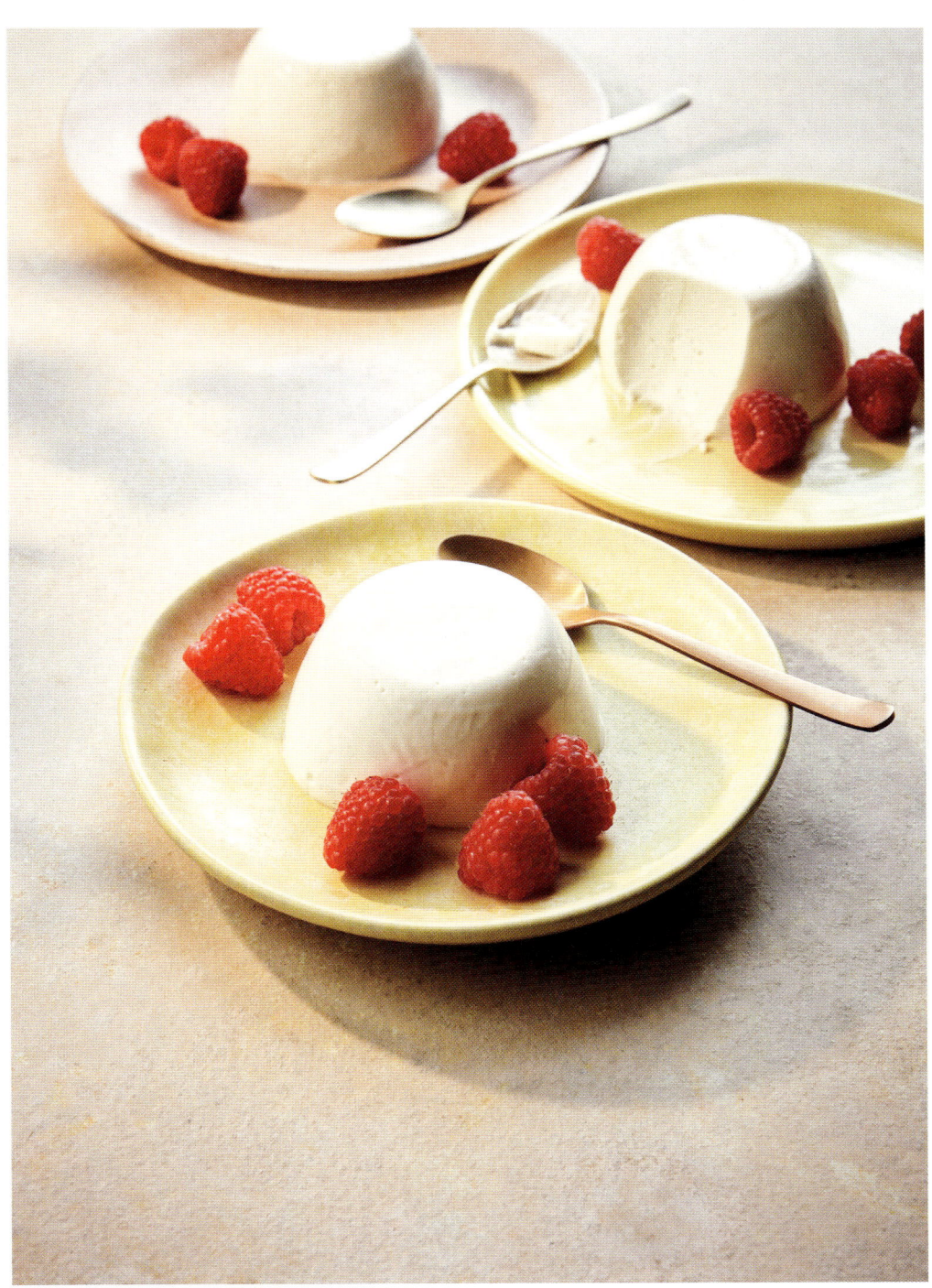

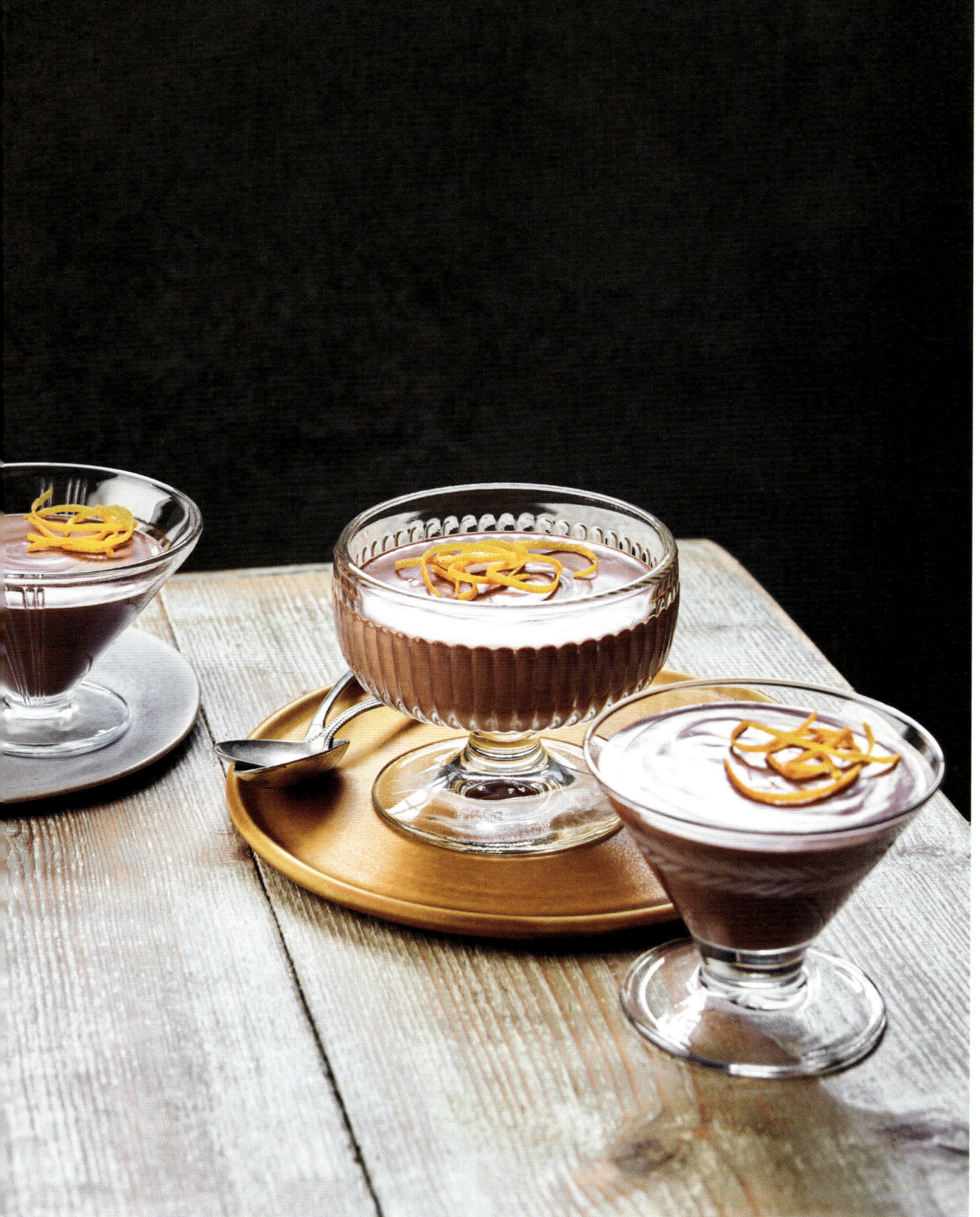

*This mousse is rich and decadent, yet it is a source of lovely antioxidants and protein. It is intense, creamy and infused with a hint of orange, making it a perfect treat to satisfy a sweet tooth. High in protein, it's definitely worth a try for a healthy dessert.*

# Dark Chocolate Orange Silken Tofu Pots

**MAKES 6 SMALL POTS OR 4 LARGE**
**Under 238kcal (4 pots), 7g protein per serving**

100g (3½oz) dark chocolate, 70% cocoa solids, chopped

300g (10½oz) silken tofu, drained

1 tablespoon unsweetened cocoa powder

3 tablespoons maple syrup or honey

Zest of 1 orange, plus extra (optional) to decorate

1 teaspoon vanilla extract

Pinch of salt

Melt the chocolate in a heatproof bowl set over a pan of simmering water, making sure the bottom of the bowl isn't touching the water, stirring occasionally until smooth. Alternatively, melt the chocolate in the microwave in 30-second intervals, stirring between each interval until fully melted.

In a blender or food processor, combine the drained tofu, melted chocolate, cocoa powder, maple syrup or honey, orange zest, vanilla extract and salt. Blend until the mixture is completely smooth and creamy. Taste and adjust the sweetness if needed by adding more maple syrup or honey.

Divide the mousse evenly between 6 small pots or 4 larger pots. Refrigerate for at least 1 hour to allow the mousse to set.

Decorate with orange zest, if you like, before serving.

*This cake is packed with thinly sliced apples and warm cinnamon, creating a deliciously moist and healthy bake. It is sweetened with honey and made with a light custard-like batter. Enjoy the cake warmed with a dollop of yogurt for a comforting and satisfying treat.*

# Layered Spiced Apple Cake

**SERVES 6**
**Under 195kcal,**
**6g protein per serving**

3 medium free-range
  eggs, lightly beaten
160ml (⅔ cup) milk
3 tablespoons extra
  virgin olive oil
1 teaspoon vanilla extract
70g (generous ½ cup) plain
  (all-purpose) flour
3 tablespoons honey
1 teaspoon ground cinnamon
Pinch of salt
4 dessert apples (skin on)
1 teaspoon baking powder

Preheat the oven to 180°C/160°C fan (350°F) Gas Mark 4. Line a 900g (2lb) loaf tin (pan) with nonstick baking paper.

In a large bowl, whisk together the eggs, milk, olive oil, vanilla extract, flour, honey, cinnamon and salt until smooth. Set aside.

Using a mandoline or the slicer side of a grater, thinly slice the apples, discarding the cores. The slices need to be very thin for the recipe to work properly.

Add the baking powder to the batter and mix well. Fold in the thin apple slices, ensuring they are evenly coated with the batter.

Tip the apple slices and batter mixture into the prepared loaf tin, pressing down to ensure there are no air pockets. Pour any remaining batter over the top and pat down to compact the mixture.

Bake in the oven for 50 minutes, or until the top is golden brown and a skewer inserted into the centre comes out clean. Be careful to watch the cake towards the end of the baking time to prevent burning.

Allow the cake to rest in the tin a little before turning it out on to a wire rack to cool completely.

Store the cake in the refrigerator, where it will keep well for up to 5 days. When ready to serve, cut a slice and warm it in a pan on either side until caramelised. Serve with a dollop of yogurt.

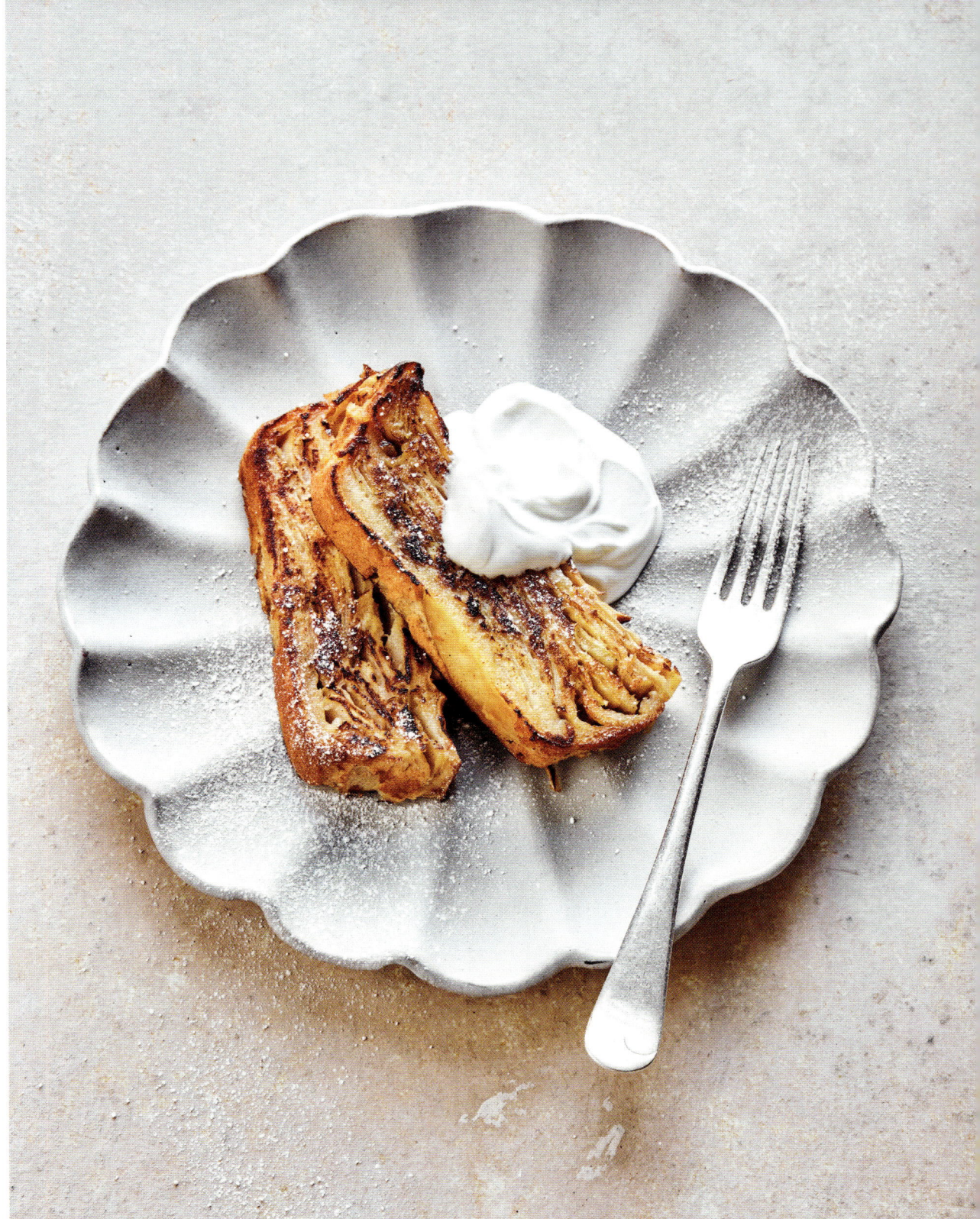

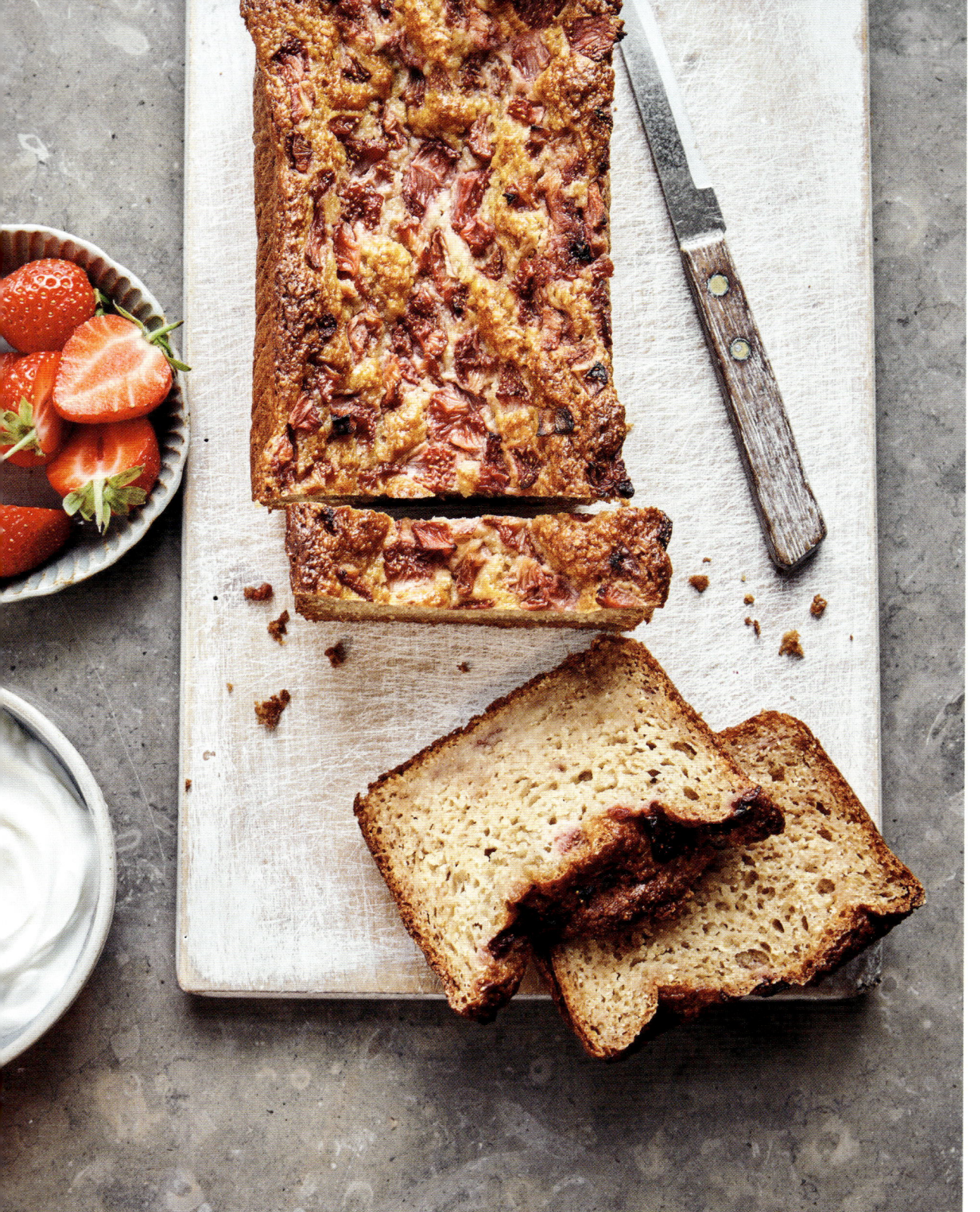

*This breakfast loaf contains a whole tub of strawberry yogurt to give it the most delicious, moist crumb as well as packing it with protein and flavour, combined with high-fibre oat flour and ground almonds. Bake into muffins for ease if you don't have a large enough loaf tin.*

# Strawberry Shortcake Yogurt Breakfast Loaf

**MAKES 10 SLICES**
**Under 210kcal,**
**9g protein per serving**

450g (scant 2 cups)
Skyr-style strawberry
yogurt (I use Arla)

2 large free-range eggs, at
room temperature

1 teaspoon vanilla extract

100g (½ cup) caster (superfine)
sugar (or a granulated
sweetener replacement)

Zest of ½ lemon

1 tablespoon extra
virgin olive oil

1 teaspoon bicarbonate
of soda (baking soda)

2 teaspoons baking powder

150g (5½oz) oat flour
or ground oats

50g (6 tablespoons) plain
(all-purpose) flour

50g (½ cup) ground almonds

Cupped handful of
strawberries, diced

Preheat the oven to 190°C/170°C fan (375°F) Gas Mark 5. Line a 900g (2lb) loaf tin (pan) with nonstick baking paper (no need to line if the loaf tin is nonstick).

In a bowl, mix the yogurt with the eggs, vanilla extract, sugar, lemon zest and olive oil, until smooth. Fold in the bicarb and baking powder, then the oat and plain flour and the ground almonds. Do not over-mix the batter. Tip into the lined tin and sprinkle the diced strawberries over the top.

Bake for 50–60 minutes until a skewer inserted into the centre comes out clean, watching to ensure it doesn't burn (cover the cake with foil if it starts to brown too quickly). Everyone's oven varies slightly, so check, and if needed, bake for an additional 15 minutes. Allow to rest for 15 minutes before serving.

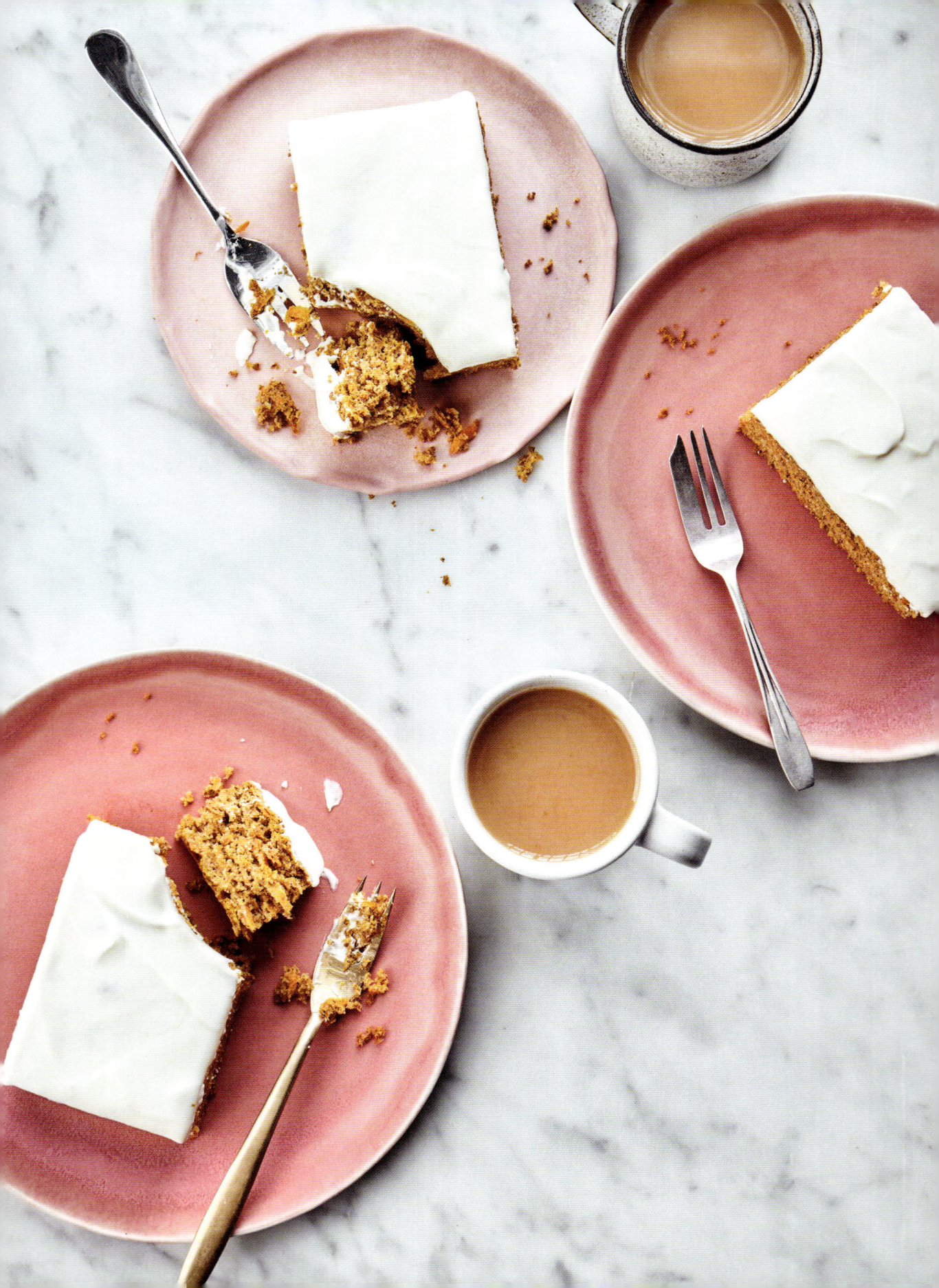

*This healthy cake is full of grated carrots, wholemeal flour and ground almonds. Topped with a silky maple cream cheese icing, this is rich, moist and absolutely delicious.*

# Carrot Cake with Maple Cream Cheese Frosting

**MAKES 10 SLICES**
**Under 265kcal,**
**5g protein per serving**

140g (⅔ cup) dates, pitted
¼ teaspoon bicarbonate of soda (baking soda)
100g wholemeal (wholewheat) flour
2 teaspoons baking powder
2 teaspoons ground cinnamon
¼ teaspoon ground nutmeg
¼ teaspoon ground ginger
100g (1 cup) jumbo oats
2 large free-range eggs
150ml (⅔ cup) olive oil
2 tablespoons brown sugar
3 tablespoons milk
Zest of 1 orange
180g (1½ cups) grated carrots
50g (1¾oz) mixed nuts, chopped and roasted

**FOR THE MAPLE CREAM CHEESE FROSTING**
250g (1 cup) light cream cheese
4 tablespoons maple syrup
1 teaspoon vanilla extract

Preheat the oven to 200°C/180°C fan (400°F) Gas Mark 6. Line a baking tin (pan), about 23 x 33cm (9 x 13 inches), with nonstick baking paper.

Place the pitted dates in a small bowl. Cover them with boiling water and add the bicarbonate of soda. Let them soak for 10 minutes, until softened. Drain the dates, and then mash or blend into a paste.

In a large bowl, whisk together the wholemeal flour, baking powder, cinnamon, nutmeg, ginger and oats. Mix well to combine.

In a separate bowl, whisk the eggs. Stir in the olive oil, brown sugar, mashed dates, milk and orange zest. Mix until smooth.

Gradually fold the wet ingredients into the dry ingredients. Add the grated carrot and chopped nuts, stirring until just combined.

Pour the batter into the prepared baking tin and spread it out evenly. Bake for 25–30 minutes, or until a toothpick inserted into the centre comes out clean. Allow the cake to cool completely in the tin.

In a medium bowl, beat the cream cheese until smooth. Add the maple syrup and vanilla extract, mixing until creamy.

Once the cake has cooled, spread the frosting evenly over the top. Cut into 10 slices and serve.

*This upside-down cake is a show-stopper dessert that combines the sweetness of fresh mangos with a rich miso caramel glaze. The almond yogurt cake batter ensures a moist and tender crumb, while the Greek yogurt adds a boost of protein. Perfect for any special occasion.*

# Mango Upside-down Cake with Almond, Yogurt and Miso Caramel

**SERVES 10**
**Under 560kcal,**
**9.3g protein per serving**

2 ripe mangos, peeled,
  pitted and sliced, plus
  extra (optional) to serve
150g (1¼ cups) self-raising
  (self-rising) flour
100g (1 cup) ground almonds
165g (¾ cup) unsalted butter
75g (⅓ cup) natural yogurt
200g (1 cup) golden caster
  (superfine) sugar
3 large free-range eggs
Zest of 1 lime
Olive oil, for greasing

**FOR THE MISO CARAMEL**
100g (½ cup) light brown sugar
60g (¼ cup) unsalted butter
2 tablespoons white
  miso paste
2 tablespoons water

Preheat the oven to 180°C/160°C fan (350°F) Gas Mark 4. Grease a 23cm (9 inch) round cake tin (pan) with a little oil.

In a small saucepan, combine the miso caramel ingredients and place over a low to medium heat for 5–10 minutes, until bubbling and slightly thickened, then stir occasionally until smooth and the sugar has dissolved.

Pour the miso caramel into the prepared cake tin, spreading it evenly across the base. Arrange the mango slices on top of the caramel in an even layer.

In a large bowl, whisk together the flour and ground almonds. In another bowl, whisk together the butter, yogurt, sugar, eggs and lime zest until smooth and well combined. Gradually add the wet ingredients to the dry ingredients, mixing until just combined. Be careful not to over-mix. Pour the batter over the mango slices, smoothing the top.

Bake in the oven for 40–50 minutes, or until a toothpick inserted into the centre of the cake comes out clean. Allow the cake to cool in the tin for 10 minutes, then carefully invert on to a serving plate. Allow the cake to cool completely before serving.

Slice and serve the cake with additional fresh mango slices, or a dollop of Greek yogurt, if desired.

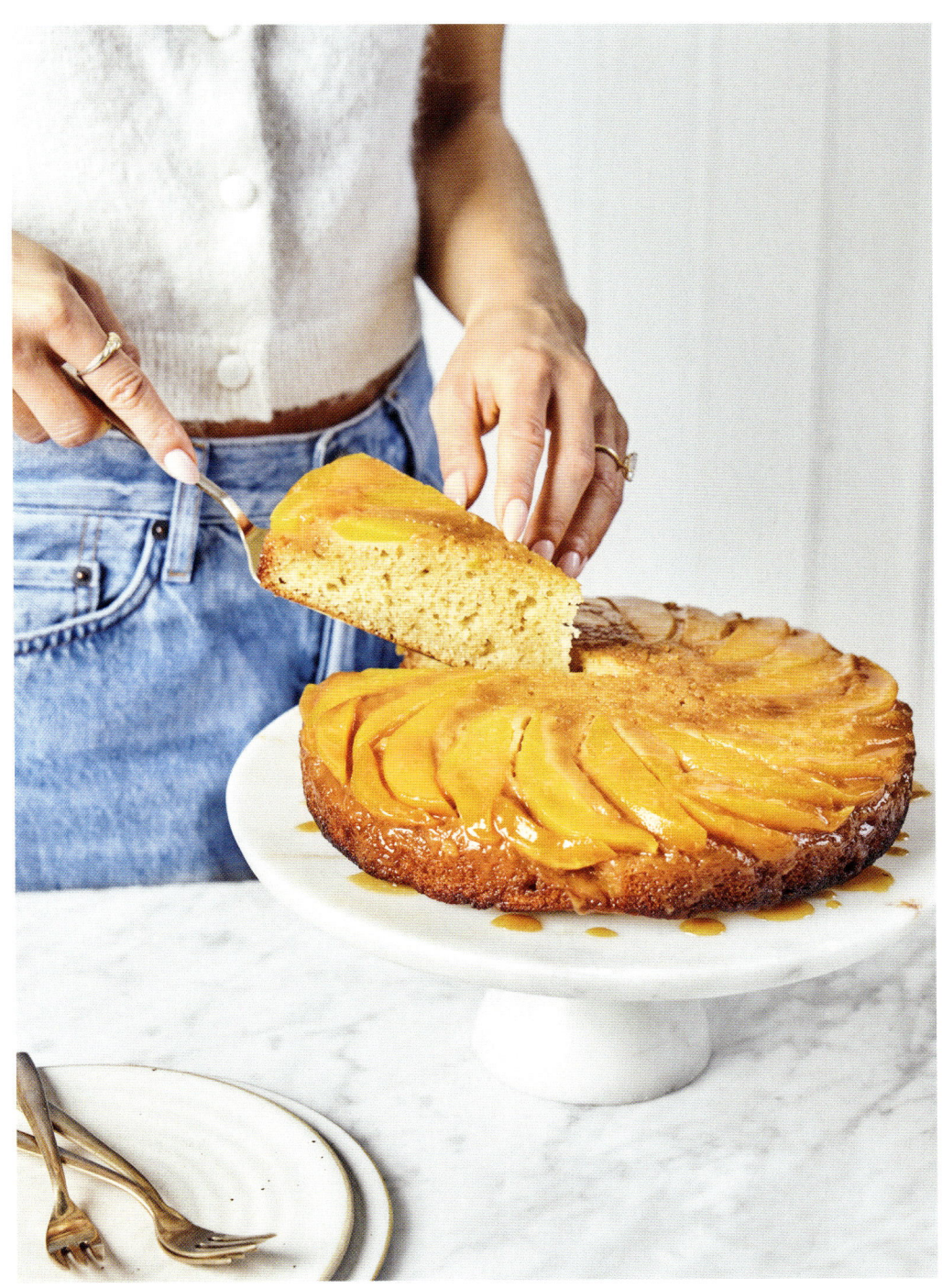

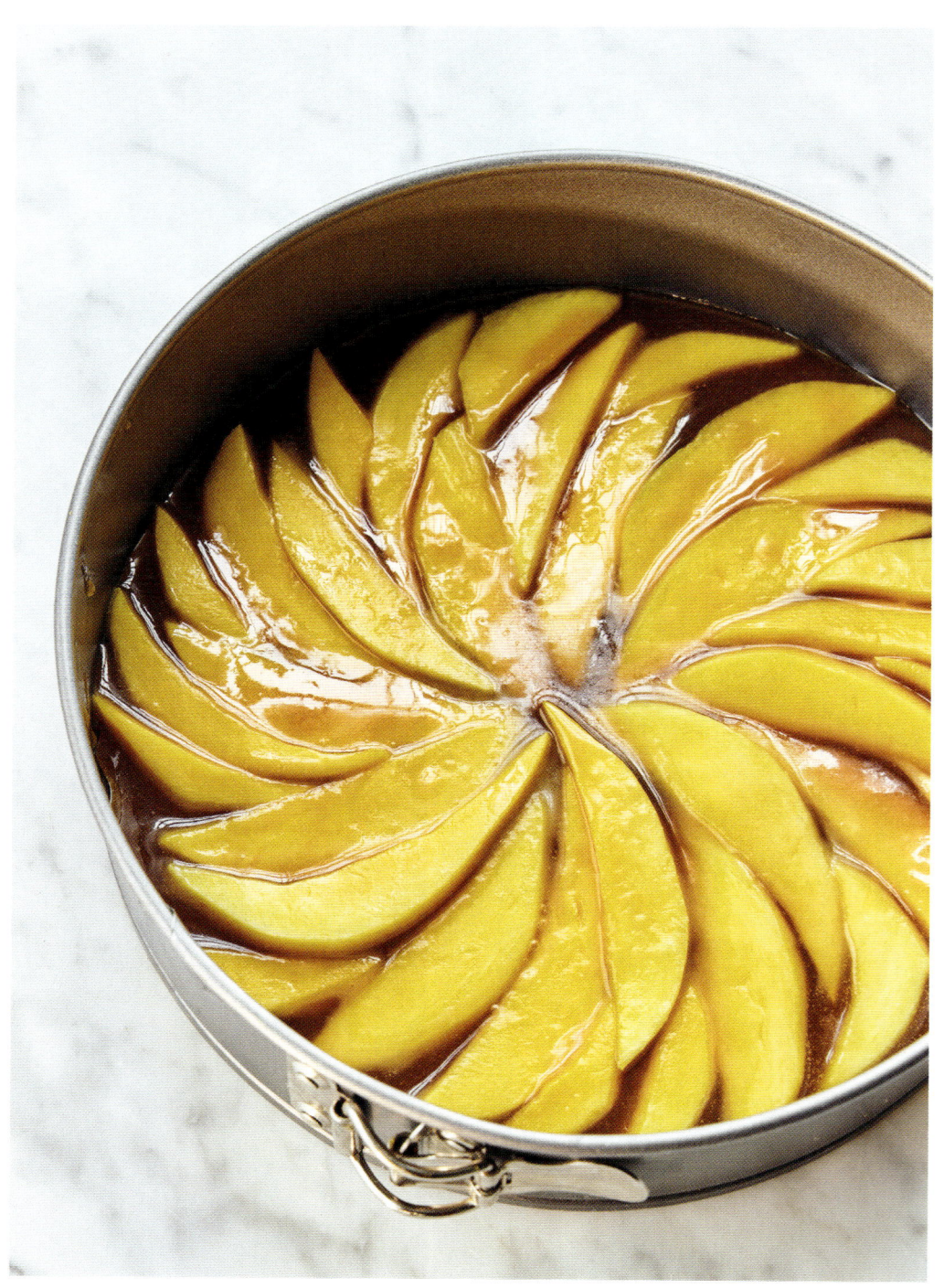

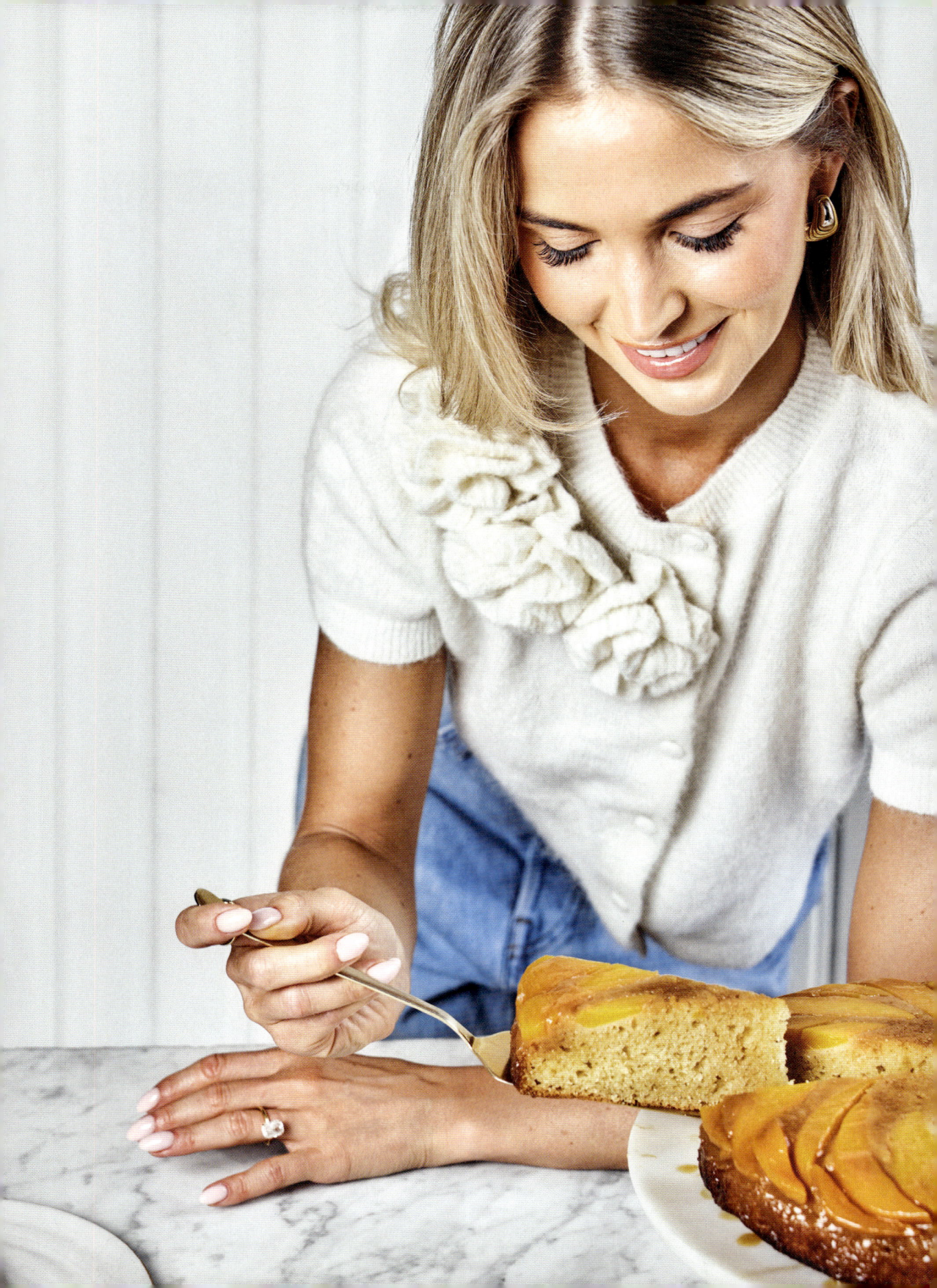

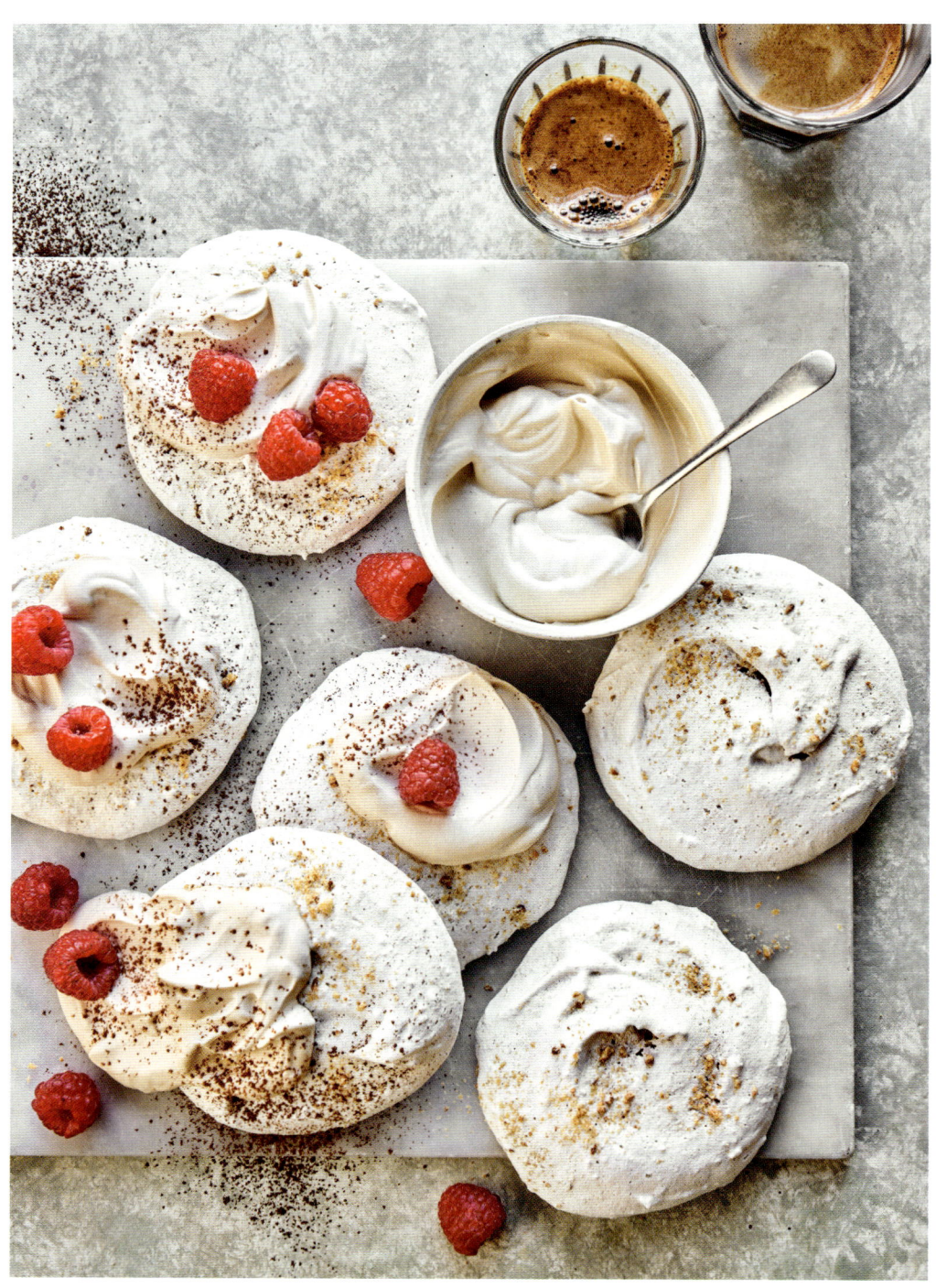

*These delightful hazelnut meringues are light and crispy, paired with a healthier, lighter coffee cream; perfect for a sophisticated dessert or a special treat. This recipe is a family favourite – they were always on the menu at my granny's restaurant.*

# Granny's Hazelnut Meringues with Light Coffee Cream

**SERVES 6**
**Under 350kcal,**
**6g protein per serving**

100g (¾ cup) hazelnuts
3 large free-range egg whites
170g (¾ cup plus 1½ tablespoons) caster (superfine) sugar or demerara (turbinado) sugar
Raspberries, to serve

**FOR THE LIGHT COFFEE CREAM**
100ml (scant ½ cup) double (heavy) cream
100g (scant ½ cup) Greek yogurt (0% or 5% fat)
2 tablespoons honey or maple syrup
2 teaspoons instant coffee granules, dissolved in 1 tablespoon hot water, then cooled
1 teaspoon vanilla extract

Preheat the oven to 140°C/120°C fan (275°F) Gas Mark 1. Line a baking tray with nonstick baking paper.

Spread the hazelnuts on a baking sheet and toast in the oven for about 8–10 minutes or until golden brown and fragrant. Remove from the oven and let them cool slightly. Rub them in a tea (dish) towel to remove the skins. Place the hazelnuts in a food processor and pulse until finely chopped, but not too much; they should still have some texture.

In a clean, dry bowl, whisk the egg whites using an electric mixer until soft peaks form. Gradually add the sugar, a tablespoon at a time, while continuing to whisk, until they form stiff, glossy peaks. Gently fold in most of the chopped hazelnuts, being careful not to over-mix.

Drop spoonfuls of the meringue mixture on to the prepared baking tray to form 6 mounds, and sprinkle a little of the reserved chopped hazelnuts on top of each meringue. Bake for 1½–2 hours, or until the meringues are dry and can be easily lifted off the nonstick baking paper. Turn off the oven and let the meringues cool completely inside, with the door slightly ajar.

In a bowl, whip the cream until soft peaks form. Gently fold in the yogurt, honey or maple syrup, dissolved coffee and vanilla extract. Mix until well combined and smooth. Chill in the refrigerator until ready to serve.

Place a dollop of light coffee cream on top of each hazelnut meringue, along with some fresh raspberries.

*This healthy tiffin-inspired dessert is a delicious, no-bake sweet hit packed with wholesome ingredients like oats, nuts, dried fruits and antioxidant-rich dark chocolate. It provides a satisfying crunch and a burst of natural sweetness.*

# Toasted Oat Chocolate Tiffin

**MAKES 16 SQUARES**
**Under 185kcal,**
**5g protein per serving**

100g (1 cup) jumbo oats

50g (1¾oz) mixed nuts (almonds, walnuts, pecans), chopped

2 tablespoons chia seeds or flaxseeds

50g (½ cup) ground almonds

50g (1¾oz) dried fruit (raisins, cranberries, apricots), chopped

2 tablespoons unsweetened cocoa powder

100g (3½oz) dark chocolate, 70% cocoa solids, broken into pieces, plus 50g (1¾oz), melted, for drizzling

100g (scant ½ cup) natural peanut butter or almond butter

4 tablespoons honey or maple syrup

1 teaspoon vanilla extract

Pinch of salt

Preheat the oven to 200°C/180°C fan (400°F) Gas Mark 6. Line a 20cm (8 inch) square baking tin (pan) or dish with nonstick baking paper.

Spread the oats, nuts and seeds on a large baking sheet and toast in the oven for about 8 minutes, checking often, until the oats are crispy and the nuts are lightly browned. Tip on to a plate and leave to cool a little.

In a large bowl, combine the ground almonds, dried fruit and cocoa powder. Add the cooled toasted oat, nut and seed mixture, then mix well to ensure even distribution.

In a microwave-safe bowl, gently melt the chocolate, peanut butter or almond butter, honey or maple syrup, vanilla extract and salt in 30-second intervals in the microwave, stirring between each interval until smooth and well combined.

Pour the melted mixture over the dry ingredients. Mix thoroughly until all the dry ingredients are well coated. Tip into the lined baking tin and press the mixture firmly, ensuring it is evenly spread and compact.

Refrigerate the tiffin for at least 2 hours or until firm and set. In a microwave-safe bowl, gently melt the remaining chocolate and drizzle it over the top of the set tiffin.

Once the chocolate has set, remove the tiffin from the baking tin and cut it into 16 squares. Serve immediately or store in an airtight container in the refrigerator for up to a week.

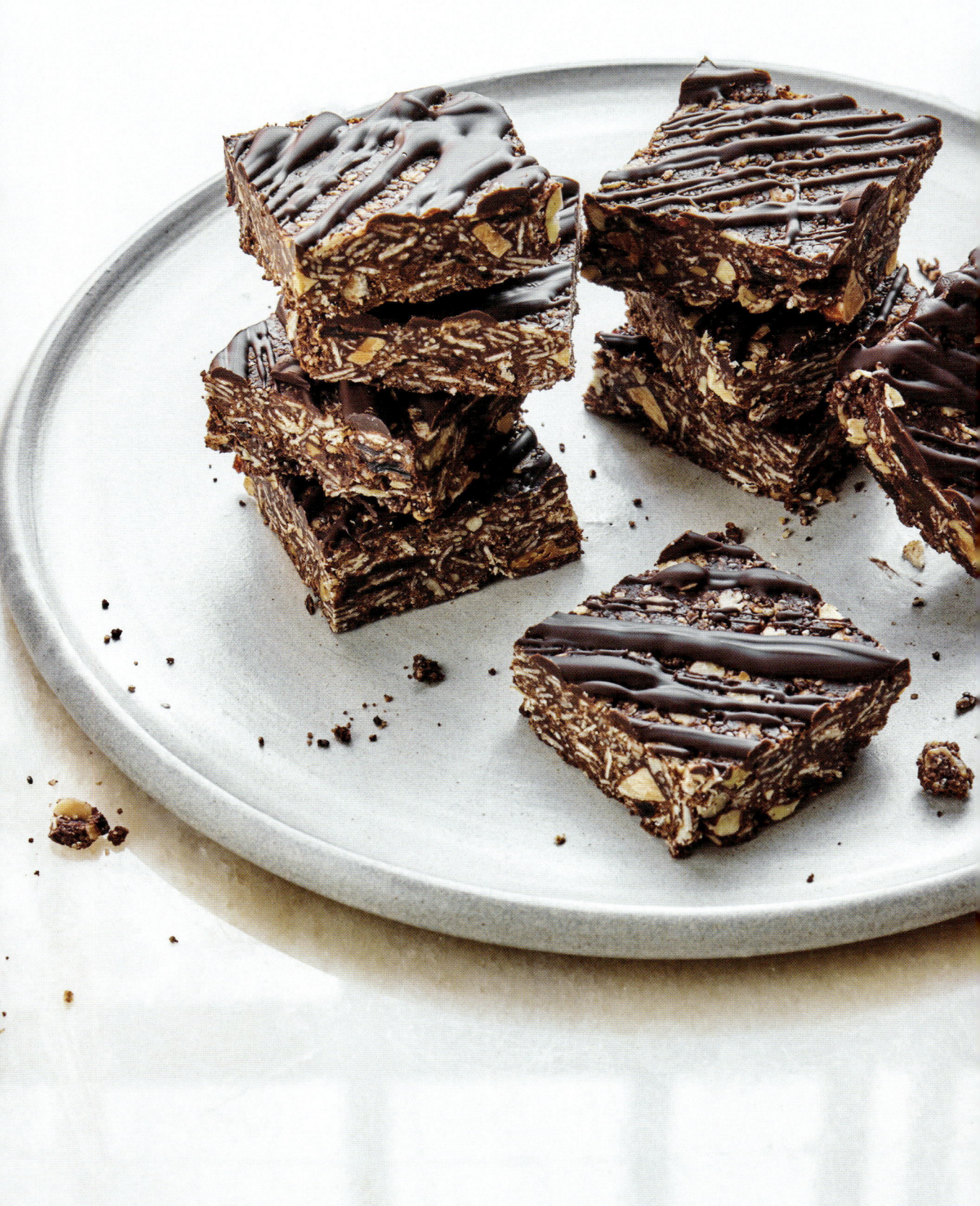

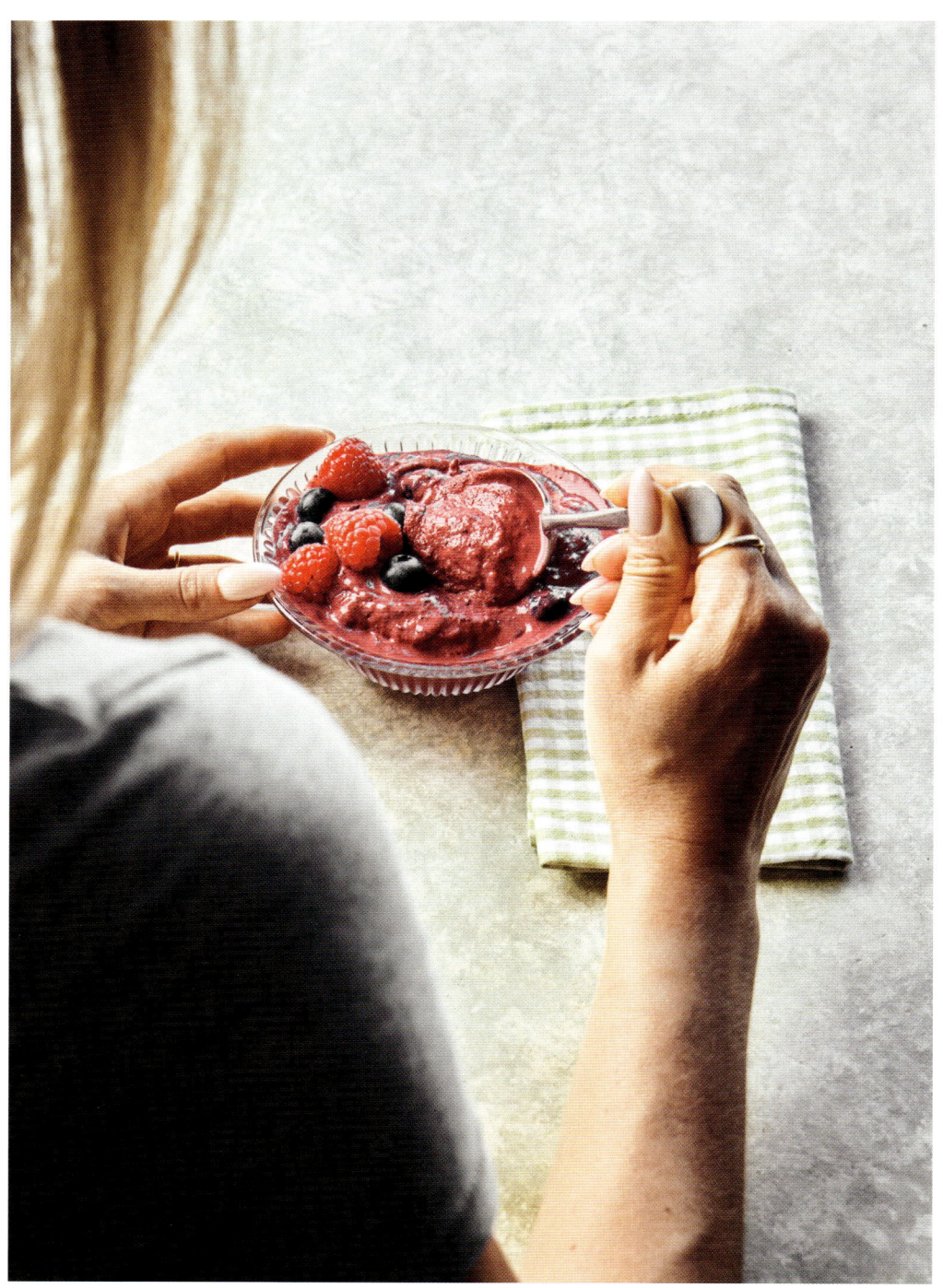

*This instant frozen berry yogurt is a quick, healthy and delicious single-serve dessert or snack. It's perfect for satisfying a sweet tooth, packed with antioxidants and protein that support good gut health, blood sugar control and will keep you full and satisfied. Use any frozen fruits you like!*

# Instant Frozen Berry Yogurt

**SERVES 1**
**Under 150kcal,**
**12g protein per serving**

150g (5½oz) frozen mixed berries, or any frozen fruits of choice

100g (scant ½ cup) Greek yogurt (0% or full fat)

1–2 teaspoons honey or maple syrup (optional, to taste)

½ teaspoon vanilla extract (optional)

Place all the ingredients in a blender or food processor and blend on high until the mixture is smooth and creamy. You may need to stop and scrape down the sides of the blender or processor to ensure everything is well combined.

Transfer the frozen berry yogurt to a bowl and enjoy immediately for the best texture.

# Meal Plans

# Meal Plans

## WHEN YOU'RE MAKING MEAL PLANS, THINK ABOUT THE FOLLOWING:

**Food Diversity:** Eating a variety of foods is essential for supporting our gut health. This meal plan shows you how to maximise food diversity to support your overall well-being.

**Meal Prep:** Choose dinner recipes that can also serve as the next day's lunch to simplify meal prep and save time.

**Oily Fish:** It is generally recommended to consume at least two portions of fish per week, of which at least one should be oily fish. Oily fish is high in omega-3 fatty acids, which are beneficial for heart health.

**Protein Flexibility:** Feel free to swap proteins in recipes according to your preference. If a recipe calls for chicken, you're welcome to use another protein source to suit your preferences or swap in a high-protein legume or tofu to go veggie.

**Cooking Flexibility:** You don't have to cook from scratch every day. Use the meal plan as a guideline for balancing your meals, and adjust as needed for your lifestyle.

I've left you some space to write out your own meals plans for the coming weeks, so you can tailor them to your preferences and lifestyle. Use these tips and the meal plan opposite as a basic guide to help you structure your main meals, and feel free to add in snacks or sweets to suit you.

## DAY 1

**Breakfast:** Cottage Cheese and Oat Protein Pancakes

**Lunch:** BLT Pasta Salad

**Dinner:** Longevity Minestrone

## DAY 2

**Breakfast:** Breakfast Bruschetta

**Lunch:** Sticky Cashew Orange Slaw

**Dinner:** Crab, Chilli and Courgette Spaghetti

## DAY 3

**Breakfast:** Herby Fluffy Folded Eggs

**Lunch:** Spicy Chicken Crunch Bagels

**Dinner:** Baked Salmon with Sauce Vierge

## DAY 4

**Breakfast:** Apple Crumble Oat Pots

**Lunch:** Tomato Tarts with Herby Feta and Ricotta

**Dinner:** Crispy Potato Fish Pie Bake

## DAY 5

**Breakfast:** Super Beans on Toast

**Lunch:** Hot Smoked Salmon Potato Salad with Citrus Vinaigrette

**Dinner:** Yogurt Harissa Chicken with Smoky Rice

## DAY 6

**Breakfast:** Tiramisu-inspired Granola

**Lunch:** Halloumi Sweet Potato Jackets with Basil Yogurt

**Dinner:** Sticky Orange and Cashew Chicken Bowls

## DAY 7

**Breakfast:** Balsamic Mushroom Stuffed Omelette

**Lunch:** Crispy Smashed Potato Mackerel Salad

**Dinner:** Whipped Ricotta and Slow-roasted Tomato Gnocchi

|                     | DAY 1 | DAY 2 | DAY 3 |
|---------------------|-------|-------|-------|
| BREAKFAST           |       |       |       |
| LUNCH               |       |       |       |
| DINNER              |       |       |       |
| SNACKS AND SWEETS   |       |       |       |

| DAY 4 | DAY 5 | DAY 6 | DAY 7 |
|-------|-------|-------|-------|
|       |       |       |       |
|       |       |       |       |
|       |       |       |       |
|       |       |       |       |

|  | DAY 1 | DAY 2 | DAY 3 |
|---|---|---|---|
| BREAKFAST |  |  |  |
| LUNCH |  |  |  |
| DINNER |  |  |  |
| SNACKS AND SWEETS |  |  |  |

| DAY 4 | DAY 5 | DAY 6 | DAY 7 |
|-------|-------|-------|-------|
|       |       |       |       |
|       |       |       |       |
|       |       |       |       |
|       |       |       |       |

# Index &
# Conversions

# Index

# Conversions

Below are the main conversions for both metric and imperial units. I have used metric scales when designing these recipes, so I recommend following these quantities for the best accuracy.

## WEIGHT CONVERSIONS

| GRAMS | OUNCES |
| --- | --- |
| 10g | ¼oz |
| 15g | ½oz |
| 20g | ¾oz |
| 30g | 1oz |
| 40g | 1½oz |
| 50g | 1¾oz |
| 60g | 2¼oz |
| 70g | 2½oz |
| 80g | 2¾oz |
| 90g | 3¼oz |
| 100g | 3½oz |
| 150g | 5½oz |
| 200g | 7oz |
| 250g | 9oz |
| 300g | 10½oz |
| 350g | 12oz |
| 400g | 14oz |
| 450g | 1lb |
| 500g | 1lb 2oz |

## VOLUME CONVERSIONS

| MILLILITRES | FLUID OUNCES |
| --- | --- |
| 50ml | 2fl oz |
| 80ml | 2¾fl oz |
| 100ml | 3½fl oz |
| 125ml | 4fl oz |
| 150ml | 5¼fl oz |
| 175ml | 6fl oz |
| 200ml | 7fl oz |
| 225ml | 8fl oz |
| 250ml | 9fl oz |
| 275ml | 9½fl oz |
| 300ml | 10½fl oz |
| 350ml | 12fl oz |
| 400ml | 14fl oz |
| 450ml | 16fl oz |
| 500ml | 18fl oz |
| 750ml | 26½fl oz |
| 1 litre | 35fl oz |

## LIQUIDS

| SPOONS & CUPS | MILLILITRES |
| --- | --- |
| ½ teaspoon | 2.5ml |
| 1 teaspoon | 5ml |
| 1 tablespoon | 15ml |
| ¼ cup | 60ml |
| ⅓ cup | 80ml |
| ½ cup | 125ml |
| 1 cup | 250ml |

## OVEN TEMPERATURES

| GAS MARK | CELSIUS | FAHRENHEIT |
| --- | --- | --- |
| 1 | 140°C | 275°F |
| 2 | 150°C | 300°F |
| 3 | 160°C | 325°F |
| 4 | 180°C | 350°F |
| 5 | 190°C | 375°F |
| 6 | 200°C | 400°F |
| 7 | 220°C | 425°F |
| 8 | 230°C | 450°F |
| 9 | 250°C | 475°F |
| 10 | 260°C | 500°F |

# Acknowledgements

To my incredible audience: thank you from the bottom of my heart. This book is for you and because of you. Each recipe here is a celebration of our shared love for delicious, nutritious food, and nothing makes me happier than seeing these meals become a part of your lives. For everyone who has made my recipes, shared them, and offered your thoughts and support – you've turned this passion into something greater than I could have ever dreamt.

It's always been my goal to create recipes that are both nourishing and tasty – the food you WANT to eat, designed by a nutritionist. Knowing that these dishes have helped to make your days a little brighter, healthier and happier means the world to me.

Thank you for trusting me to bring these recipes into your kitchens and for letting me be a part of your journey to a balanced, joy-filled life. Here's to many more meals, memories and moments shared across our tables.

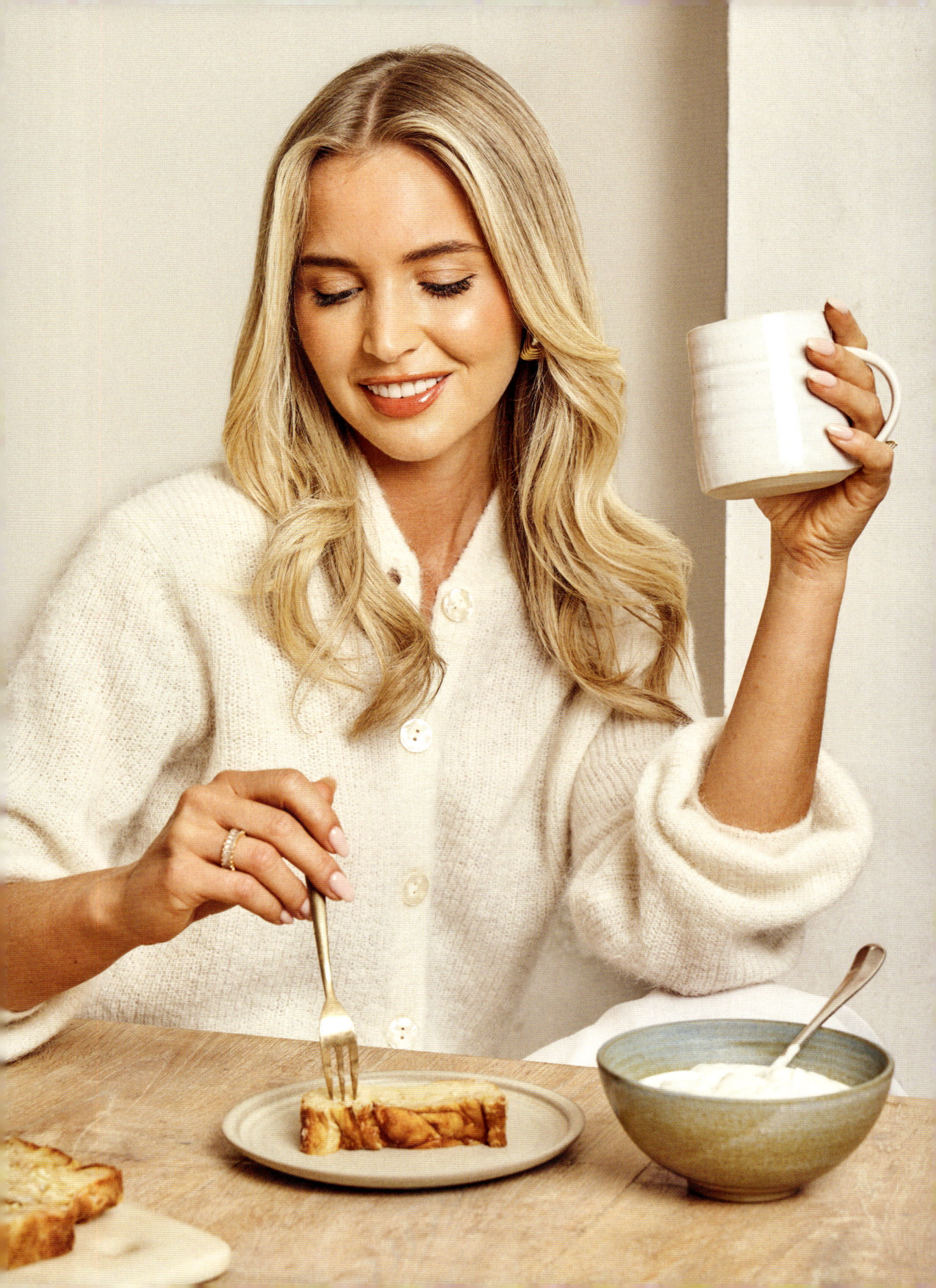

# Credits

**Publisher**
Vicky Eribo

**Senior
Commissioning Editor**
George Brooker

**Copy-editor**
Sally Somers

**Proofreader**
Kate Truman

**Indexer**
Ingrid Lock

**Editorial Management**
Susie Bertinshaw
Jane Hughes
Charlie Panayiotou
Lucy Bilton
Patrice Nelson

**Contracts**
Dan Herron
Ellie Bowker
Oliver Chacón

**Design**
Nick Shah
Deborah Francois

**Art Direction**
Helen Ewing
Hart Studio

**Cover Design**
Jessica Hart

**Interior Design**
Hart Studio

**Photo Shoots &
Image Research**
Natalie Dawkins

**Photographer**
Clare Winfield

**Food and
Props Stylist**
Libby Silbermann

**Food Stylist Assistant**
Florence Blair

**Hair Stylist**
Sarrah Hammid

**Macros**
Libby Adler

**Finance**
Nick Gibson
Jasdip Nandra
Sue Baker
Tom Costello

**Inventory**
Jo Jacobs
Dan Stevens

**Production**
Claire Keep
Katie Horrocks

**Marketing**
Corinne Jean-Jacques
Louis Patel

**Publicity**
Ellen Turner

**Sales**
David Murphy
Victoria Laws
Esther Waters
Tolu Ayo-Ajala
Group Sales teams
across Digital, Field,
International and
Non-Trade

**Operations**
Group Sales
Operations team

**Rights**
Rebecca Folland
Tara Hiatt
Ben Fowler
Alice Cottrell
Ruth Blakemore
Marie Henckel

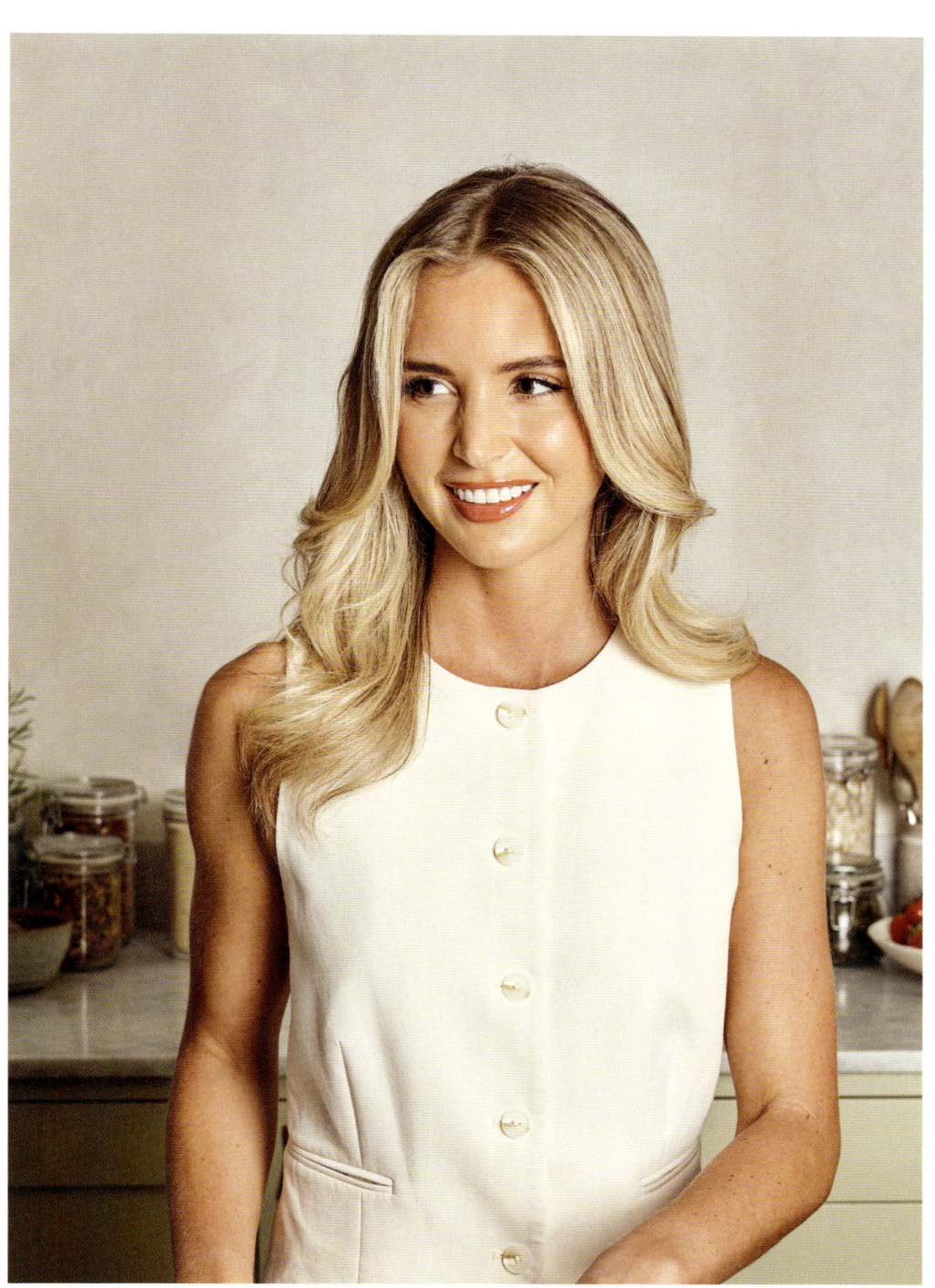

First published in Great Britain in 2025 by Seven Dials,
an imprint of The Orion Publishing Group Ltd
Carmelite House, 50 Victoria Embankment
London EC4Y 0DZ

An Hachette UK Company

The authorised representative in the EEA is Hachette Ireland,
8 Castlecourt Centre, Dublin 15, D15 XTP3, Ireland (email: info@hbgi.ie)

3 5 7 9 10 8 6 4 2

Copyright © Emily English 2025
Design and layout © The Orion Publishing Group 2025

The moral right of Emily English to be identified as
the author of this work has been asserted in accordance
with the Copyright, Designs and Patents Act of 1988.

All rights reserved. No part of this publication may be
reproduced, stored in a retrieval system, or transmitted
in any form or by any means, electronic, mechanical,
photocopying, recording, or otherwise, without the
prior permission of both the copyright owner and the
above publisher of this book.

Every effort has been made to ensure that the information in this book is accurate.
The information in this book may not be applicable in each individual case,
so it is advised that professional medical advice is obtained for specific health
matters and before changing any medication or dosage. Neither the publisher nor
author accepts any legal responsibility for any personal injury or other damage
or loss arising from the use of the information in this book. In addition, if you are
concerned about your diet or exercise regime and wish to change them,
you should consult a health practitioner first.

A CIP catalogue record for this book is
available from the British Library.

ISBN (Hardback) 978 1 3996 2007 9
ISBN (Ebook) 978 1 3996 2008 6

Typeset by Hart Studio
Printed in Italy by Printer Trento

MIX
Paper | Supporting
responsible forestry
FSC® C104740

FSC
www.fsc.org